REIKI

Self Help Guide To Cleanse Your Aura And Useful Tips For Reiki Healing and Meditation

(Increase Energy and Improve Health with Healing Energy)

Frank Stein

Published by Rob Miles

Frank Stein

All Rights Reserved

Reiki: Self Help Guide To Cleanse Your Aura And Useful Tips For Reiki Healing and Meditation (Increase Energy and Improve Health with Healing Energy)

ISBN 978-1-989990-22-3

All rights reserved. No part of this guide may be reproduced in any form without permission in writing from the publisher except in the case of brief quotations embodied in critical articles or reviews.

Legal & Disclaimer

The information contained in this book is not designed to replace or take the place of any form of medicine or professional medical advice. The information in this book has been provided for educational and entertainment purposes only.

The information contained in this book has been compiled from sources deemed reliable, and it is accurate to the best of the Author's knowledge; however, the Author cannot guarantee its accuracy and validity and cannot be held liable for any errors or omissions. Changes are periodically made to this book. You must consult your doctor or get professional medical advice before using any of the suggested remedies, techniques, or information in this book.

Upon using the information contained in this book, you agree to hold harmless the Author from and against any damages, costs, and expenses, including any legal fees potentially resulting from the application of any of the information provided by this guide. This disclaimer applies to any damages or injury caused by the use and application, whether directly or indirectly, of any advice or information presented, whether for breach of contract, tort, negligence, personal injury, criminal intent, or under any other cause of action.

You agree to accept all risks of using the information presented inside this book. You need to consult a professional medical practitioner in order to ensure you are both able and healthy enough to participate in this program.

Table of Contents

INTRODUCTION 1

CHAPTER 1: THE HISTORY OF REIKI 3

CHAPTER 2: HOW DOES REIKI WORK? 23

CHAPTER 3: WHAT IS REIKI TECHNIQUE? 29

CHAPTER 4: WHAT IS REIKI? 45

CHAPTER 5: WHAT IS REIKI? 58

CHAPTER 6: UNDERSTANDING REIKI 63

CHAPTER 7: REIKI SYMBOLS 69

CHAPTER 8: THE SENSATION OF REIKI 74

CHAPTER 9: WHY OFFER REIKI TO CATS? 83

CHAPTER 10: THE IMPORTANCE OF INITIATION SIZE 87

CHAPTER 11: THE PRINCIPLES OF REIKI.......................... 110

CHAPTER 12: HEAL YOUR EMOTIONAL AND MENTAL HEALTH 124

CHAPTER 13: IMAGINATION PLAYTIME (IT'S NOT JUST FOR KIDS) 140

CHAPTER 14: REIKI AND ALSO THE MOOD 151

CHAPTER 15: WHAT IS ENERGY HEALING? 157

CHAPTER 16: HOW IS HEALING EXPECTED TO BE OBTAINED FROM USING THIS MEDICATION TECHNIQUES? 164

CHAPTER 17: LEARNING TO PRACTICE REIKI 174

CONCLUSION 182

Introduction

Reiki is a type of alternative therapy commonly known as energy cure. It was established in Japan in the late 1800s, and the universal energy from the hands of the practitioner to his patient is said to be transferred.

Power healing has been used in various forms for centuries. Advocates say that it interacts with the body's energy fields.

Reiki is somewhat controversial because it is difficult to prove its effectiveness through scientific means. But many people who receive Reiki claim that it works and its popularity is growing. Google's word quest currently returns no less than 68,900,000 results.

A survey conducted in 2007 shows that 1.2 million adults in the United States tried Reiki or similar therapy at least once in the preceding year. It is estimated that more than 60 hospitals offer Reiki services to patients.

Fast facts on Reiki

Here are some of Reiki's key points. More details can be found in the main book.

• Reiki is an energy therapy form.

• Notwithstanding skepticism in some quarters, interest is increasing.

• It involves energy transfer by hand laying.

• Reiki advocates say many conditions and emotional states can be treated.

• Small studies indicate that Reiki can reduce pain significantly, but no studies show that it is effective in the treatment of any disease.

• Reiki offers some hospitals in the USA and Europe, but insurance seldom covers it.

Chapter 1: The History Of Reiki

What is Reiki?

Reiki is a form of therapy that promotes healing and balance in life.

The practice of Reiki improves relaxation and reduces stress, both of which are prevalent in society.

The focus of Reiki is to improve or increase the flow of positive energy through the use of energy that flows from the hands of the practitioner.

The idea is to improve areas of low or weak energy, which are considered areas of illness, to improve well being.

The word Reiki originates from the Japanese words for Rei, which refers to a "higher power" or "power of the universe", spirituality, or universal power, and Ki, which refers to energy or life force.

These two words combined are defined as a spiritually guided energy, which is the definition of Reiki.

The Origin of Reiki and How the Practice has Developed

The history of Reiki dates to ancient times, though the exact era or time period is unknown.

In more recent history, between the mid-1800s and early 20th century, the practice of Reiki was rediscovered and developed for modern use, as it is applied today.

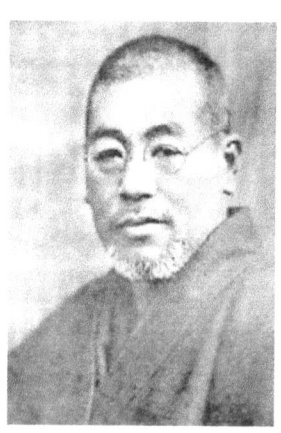

Dr. Usai, a Buddhist monk from Japan, studied the ancient practice, discovering its benefits and developing Reiki further to enhance the benefits on a spiritual, mental and physical level.

In just over a century, Reiki is performed all over the world, from its roots in Japan to many countries across the globe, including western countries.

While many people may use Western-based medicine and treatments for a variety of illnesses and chronic conditions, many people also look towards Reiki and other forms of healing to strengthen their mind, body, and spirituality through this practice.

How does Reiki develop?

Reiki is developed through training sessions or classes, and a series of attunements.

There is a total of three levels of study in Reiki, which provides the foundation for understanding its healing energy and how it is applied as a therapy for yourself and others.

Each level contains at least one session of attunement, which is a rite or process by with the Reiki master or instructor transfers energy to the students to enhance their healing power (this is discussed in more detail in chapter four).

The power of Reiki develops over time, as it helps to clear and heal the mind, allowing a stronger flow of positive energy to transfer from one place or person to another.

For each level of Reiki, the student develops a deeper understanding and connection with universal energy.

With each attunement, there is a stronger enhancement of that connection, and while just one attunement can last for an indefinite length of time, some students choose to remain longer for each level, to deepen their experience and energy, either through more practice, additional attunements, or both.

Some people new to the practice, with little or no Reiki knowledge, may choose to take the first level only, for their own benefit or self-practice.

For others, the practice of Reiki is much more, and progressing to the third or master level is done with a great deal of passion and commitment.

Different Forms of Reiki

As Reiki developed over centuries, and within recent times, several forms of the practice became popular, and are known by their specific style or name.

While all forms of Reiki are essentially the same in principle, the style and methods in which it is practiced and treatment options used vary depending on the specific type. The following types are most commonly known as the following:

Jikiden Reiki

This is the most traditional and original form of Reiki practiced today.

It's also known as Eastern Reiki, as it is closely related to the way it was initially used when first developed.

This form has changed has not changed from its initial form and aims to closely follow the original model or techniques used in ancient times.

People who practice Jikiden Reiki are most interested in remaining with the traditional methods.

Jikiden is known as the purest form of Reiki, as it has changed the least in comparison to other forms.

There are some distinct principles related to the traditional form of Reiki, known as Jikiden, including the following:

- It promotes the quick or accelerated healing process of surgical procedures and related medical techniques

- The healing process is spiritual, though it does not aim to change nor conflict with the different beliefs of other people.

In other words, it works regardless of your religion or faith. The focus is primarily on the level of energy that is channeled, which is universal and available to everyone.

- It aims to promote and heal the psychological side of addiction and related issues that stem from both psychological and physical foundations.

This may include the alleviation of depression, anxiety, and forms of stress, which can be a recurring condition on their own or related to other conditions, which can also be treated in the same way.

- Another attribute of the goal of Jikiden Reiki is the ability to soothe and comfort without feeling invasive or uncomfortable, and this is also common in all forms of Reiki.

Hands are often placed over each area to be treated, or lightly touching the area for the same effect.

- This form of Reiki also aims to correct negative habits that are self-destructive, including compulsivity and addiction or repetitive behaviors that cause grief in our lives.

For example, people prone to substance abuse and gambling would benefit from this form of Reiki

Usui Reiki

Also known as the Western method, this style of Reiki remains close to Master Miao Usui's developments, though it has been revised and changed for common versions of the practice in Western countries.

Usui worked with the original form of Reiki, making some changes to enhance its ability, which has gone through further changes since.

Both forms (Jikiden and Usui), as with all Reiki styles, are referred to as a form of spiritual healing through physical means, where the light or energy is transferred or channeled through the hands from one person to the other, for the benefit of healing and other positive effects.

The Usui form of Reiki focuses on a specific set of principles and benefits as follows:

● There is a great deal of focus on accepting yourself as is and being able to practice and enjoy the benefits of Reiki anywhere at any time.

While the practice itself involves the transference of universal energy, there is a great deal of importance placed on the individual and their ability to benefit from this process.

● Like Jikiden Reiki, there is a focus on practicing in such a way that the experience is comfortable and brings a soothing sense to your mind and body.

- Usui is used as a way to help those who have passed away to transition or move from the current (or previous) physical existence to an afterlife or spiritual existence.

- There is a goal to reduce stress, including the tension and pressure that we accumulate daily, often without noticing.

Once this stress is lifted or calmed, the results are significant, and we feel lighter, and life becomes manageable and easier to face. Other benefits with the reduction of stress include less anxiety and a sense of fear.

- Also, like the Jikiden method, there is no conflict with other people's faiths or beliefs. The idea is to heal and comfort everyone, and this is a goal for all forms of Reiki.

- We all hide how we feel at some point, and some of us habitually hide our feelings and emotions like a regular way of dealing with them.

In Reiki, some of these emotions may rise to the surface, creating an experience that is liberating, though may cause some people to feel vulnerable. It's important to note that this is a natural effect of Reiki's strength in healing not only the physical but the emotional side as well.

- Usui Reiki aims to help people who have sustained injury and/or surgical procedures to heal quickly and effectively.

It also gives them the strength to endure the healing process and coping with life following the event.

- Sleep becomes easier and more qualitative after Reiki treatment.

Some people report the ability to fall asleep quicker than previously and experience a deeper, more satisfying rest than before.

- This form of Reiki is suitable for all ages and people, which is also the case with other forms of this practice.

Karuna Reiki

This is a form of Reiki that focuses on developing a deep sense of love and spreading it to others through the practice.

While the first two forms of Reiki focus on the physical healing process, along with the spiritual, Karuna Reiki aims to use more spiritual healing as a way to treat or improve others mentally and psychologically.

Some people who practice both Usui or Jikiden Reiki and Karuna, find that Karuna is overall stronger and has the potential for healing on a deeper level.

It builds upon the knowledge and sense of wisdom we already have, which helps us heal and improve faster on all levels (mentally, psychologically, physically, and spiritually).

The main idea is the extension of love and care to yourself and the people around you.

In doing this, the energy transfer is of a higher level and can promote healing more effectively as a result.

Many of the goals associated with this form of Reiki focus on emotional healing, and other conditions or issues associated with it:

● Karuna Reiki works to clear the mind of mental clutter and allow for better learning and a stronger understanding of knowledge.

This can help develop wisdom and promote a clearer understanding of our own thoughts and emotions.

● It provides a sense of relief and comfort for people suffering from loss or grief.

It allows them to cope while navigating through the stages of grief and processing the various emotions they will experience along this journey.

There is also some relief from the emotional pain that is experienced from a loss, and through other challenges in life as well.

- There is a focus on fostering a sense of self-acceptance and love and learning to accept the characteristics of ourselves that we find less appealing and ideal.

Some people are caught up in the negative aspects of what we don't like about our bodies and personalities, that we forget or lose sight of the positive. Karuna aims to help us accept that we are valuable despite our imperfections (or perceived imperfections), which helps boost self-esteem and a sense of worth.

- Personal goals are a focus of Karuna Reiki, and this works well with the sense of deep healing and emotional strength that is fostered through this practice.

In accepting who we are and improving our own self-love, we become more capable of achieving our own personal goals, as well as work and professional milestones.

Other benefits of Karuna Reiki include further development of self-reliance and less codependency.

The overall focus on this form of Reiki is to alleviate and treat a lot of emotional disorders and inconsistencies that we all face from time to time.

For some people, this can be more challenging to treat than others, though over time, there is a great deal of improvement and confidence as a result.

Couples looking to improve their relationship and communication skills with one another, as well as with others in their lives, can benefit significantly from Karuna Reiki.

This practice works well with both Western forms of therapy (therapy and Western medicine) as well as other alternative forms for medicine or wellness.

Sekehem Reiki (also known as Sichim Reiki)

This form of Reiki is based in Egypt and is considered the extension of healing and well being from the Egyptian Goddess Sekhmet.

The form of energy used or channeled is considered vibrational and full of light, which rejects all forms of negativity and pain that are associated with it.

The main principle of this form of Reiki is to promote positivity and build a stronger sense of spirituality through the opening of chakras and delivering a strong light or healing power.

There is a renewed sense of balance and contentment with this treatment, which begins gradually, and increases to an intense level.

The effects are powerful, and many people report the effects of just one session lasting for more than several days.

Sekehem or Sichim Reiki is often used with essential oils.

The treatment focuses on healing, emotionally and mentally, from situations that cause grieving or other stressful scenarios, including marital breakdown, loss of employment and other difficult experiences in life.

One of the main effects noticed by people who receive this form of Reiki as a treatment is the draining of energy from the negative, and a sense of relief or peace that follows.

The feelings can be intense, though favorable, and soothing at once.

The main benefits of this Reiki are as follows:

● A deeper sense of awareness and focus in life. A sense of purpose is stronger, and this fosters a better sense of confidence as well.

- Promoting connections between other people in our lives and our relationships with them. Treatment can provide an opportunity to deepen these ties and help us appreciate the positive connections we have with the closest people to us.

- The deep sense of enlightenment and spirituality, including a stronger sense of inner peace and acceptance.

- Stronger and faster healing of the emotional, spiritual, and physical within ourselves.

Karuna Reiki is a powerful way to connect with nature and the universe on a spiritual level while improving our own state of well being in the process.

The growing intensity and long-lasting effects of this practice create a long-lasting effect that can be transferred to others as it benefits us, either as a practitioner, a client, or a student.

Lightarian Reiki

This form of Reiki both combines and expands the purpose of Usui and Karuna forms, focusing on a deep sense of loving energy with strong self-building goals and healing properties.

Reiki Masters practice Lightarian Reiki to improve their spiritual level and increase their level beyond, to promote stronger healing abilities by channeling more vibrational forms of energy.

There are different bands or levels of energy in Reiki, eight in total, which create a path to higher awareness and spirituality.

The Usui and Karuna forms of Reiki are concentrated with the first two bands, while the remaining six are reached through Lightarian Reiki, to connect with Ascended Masters or a higher sense of being.

During this process of moving through the different bands of energy, there is a growing sense of empowerment within, which helps create stronger sources of energy during practice on others as well as for yourself personally.

What are the main properties and benefits of Lightarian Reiki?

The following advantages can be gained through the process of Reiki meditation and self-practice, which is detailed further in this book:

- As you progress through the higher forms of energy, this will benefit clients in your practice. You'll be giving or channeling a higher form of energy for faster and stronger healing ability.

- Along with helping others, you'll notice a higher sense of personal peace and healing within.

- Growing sensitivity and awareness for further spiritual development.

All forms of Reiki are powerful and create strong channels of energy for healing and self-betterment in many ways.

The most popular form of Reiki practiced today is Usui, as his methods are easy to follow and readily practiced throughout North America.

This form of practice remains mostly traditional, with aspects of Master Usui's enhancements, which were implemented around one hundred years ago.

If you are interested in exploring other forms of Reiki in practice, a Master or instructor may be able to refer additional resources or materials to study different forms, or depending on their own experience and training; they may be able to offer helpful advice as well.

Chapter 2: How Does Reiki Work?

Reiki treatments, as practiced in major hospitals, clinics, and by individual Reiki Masters, are effectively applied in order to:

❖ Treat the symptoms and the causes of illness

❖ Promote natural self-healing of injuries

❖ Strengthen the immune system

❖ Balance the energies of your body's organs and functions, to promote wellness

❖ Release blocked or suppressed feelings, to promote emotional & spiritual peace

❖ Enhance your ability to meditate

❖ Enhance spiritual growth and self-awareness and creativity

❖ Balance your energy centers (chakras, aura) for general Well-Being, happiness, empowerment

❖ Relaxes you and reduce stress

❖ Help you love yourself more

❖ Help you love your inner child more

❖ Balance & strengthen your emotional state

❖ Promote self-power through the power of love

❖ Promotes self confidence

"Rei" means Universe, or God Consciousness. "Ki" means Chi, or Life Force Energy.

"Reiki" means, basically, the life force energy of the universe, or of God (in Japanese).The Life Force Energy of the Universe is all around us, in us, moving through us, it is us, it is God, it is the Source of everything that exists, it is our very reason for existing, it is the very energy that is life.

Quantum physics (since Einstein 100 years ago) says that everything, is ONLY pure energy, and that what we see as the physical world is ONLY an illusion. That the physical world, our body, are things that we actually create to appear the way that they do, at every moment that we look at things or ourselves.

Quantum physics has proven that we ourselves are ONLY pure energy, that the physical being that we see in the mirror is only an illusion, that we are ONLY energy. It has proven that we are composed of the same exact energy that makes up the entire universe, which is the energy of the Source of life itself. Reiki treatments focus this universal life force energy (Chi) on your body and your spiritual being, allowing you to receive additional life force energy.

This strengthens the body and your emotional state in order to promote self-healing, it reduces stress, brings emotional balance and deep peaceful relaxation. Reiki enables a better quality of life as a result. Reiki is similar to other ancient energy healing arts such as traditional Chinese acupuncture, Chi Gong, Tai Chi, Hindu Pranic Healing, and others. It is also known to be a way of gaining powerful spiritual development as well as impressive personal growth.

A Reiki Master treats the fully-clothed patient by placing his hands in 12 positions along the energy pathways and energy centers of your body which correspond to your energy system. These energy centers are called Chakras. The hand positions that are similar to some of the places of focus in acupuncture.

For a Reiki Distance healing, I place my hands in these positions on you in a virtual way, while you're on the phone with me, or while you're meditating, or even while you're sleeping. A Reiki Master does not use their human energy for healing - we channel directly from the benevolent nourishing Universal Source, the Life Force Energy of the Universe, of God.In addition to the powerful Reiki Healing techniques and symbols, use your psychic skills of vividly tapping into Source, and shamanic breathing (holotropic breathing), to strengthen the amount and the intensity of the nurturing blissfully euphoric healing energy that I channel into your being.

Chapter 3: What Is Reiki Technique?

2.1. Short history of Reiki

When I first came across Reiki as a self-healing technique, I did not know anything about it. At first I thought it was some sort of a passing fashion in the lives of people around me who wanted to be different and feel more important than other people. Somehow by coincidence, and yet as there are no coincidences, my Reiki master and teacher appeared on my doorstep looking for some help regarding her project to start up a private radio station. After having had a friendly talk for a few hours, the two of us came to the conclusion that perhaps her project would not be carried out, but that my family and I would learn Reiki and thus take a new step towards our inner selves.

My children have confidence in me, so no one asked me where we were going that weekend. The attunement into the Reiki symbols lasted from morning till night because that was how my Reiki master conducted the initiation process. Most Reiki masters use the word 'initiation' when they are writing or materializing the Reiki symbols into a person's body. However, this word 'initiation' gives a different tone to the process of transferring the symbols and of opening the energy channels. This feels as though you were passing from one religion to another, but this is not what happens when you are learning Reiki. Reiki does not change your religious beliefs; it gives you the energy needed for your life functions and it leaves your religious and other civilization acquirements within you so that you can use them at will. So, when you are learning the Reiki symbols either at the first, second or third level, you are just reaching a more intense level of energy, which you can then direct with your palms and your mind at where you want to take action. I can already hear the following question: 'Could the use of Reiki energy have negative effects on other people?' The answer is clear, yes, the use of Reiki can have effects on other people. We affect other people by the very fact we were born. First we affect our mothers and then other members of our family who cuddle us and care for us when we are still babies. Therefore, this mutual interaction is what our everyday life is made of. Clearly, we affect everything and everybody with the Reiki energy but this time we are doing it consciously. We choose how and when to have effect on other people around us, and then we take on responsibility for our actions. As a consequence, what disappears is the need to apologize for something that has happened beyond your control and your responsibility. The need to blame the outer world for what is happening to you disappears, and you take on the responsibility for your entire being. People around you perceive you as a person who knows what they are doing and how they should live their life. Day by day you are discovering new levels of freedom and simplicity in dealing with everyday obligations, thus turning your life into play and pleasure. You learn to accept the process of getting older as a change and you stop using illnesses as a means of drawing other people's attention to yourself. Reiki is growing within you and increasing your inner energy. With the help of Reiki, you are getting closer and closer to your inner self. You are entering the world of awareness and you are becoming a person with a defined life path who knows nothing about boredom, feeling of being lost, insecurity and loneliness because your inner content is changing constantly every day. You are entering the oneness with the universal mind, from which you can draw contents which encourage and support your harmonious being.

The ideological father of this technique is Japanese theologist Dr. Mikao Usui. He was born most probably around 1865 in north Japan, and died on 9 March 1926 in a small town, Fuku Jama, in the Hiroshima County. According to some sources, he did not die before 1930. He studied the life of Jesus on the Holy Mountain when, around 1915, during one of his regular daily meditations he experienced the integration with the Reiki symbols. Having felt great happiness and enthusiasm after his first insight into the symbols, Dr. Usui asked the divine energies to give him the knowledge of their use. Through every following contact with the symbols, Dr. Usui was becoming aware of their ever growing strength until he finally received the knowledge of their use, together with the insights into what this energy carried alongside.

The technique was named according to the Japanese language, where Rei stands for the outer energy and Ki for our inner energy. By connecting these two energies, a flow of energy is created within us. This flow of energy increases our inner life energy, thus putting us in balance and harmony in our surroundings. The Reiki energy flows downwards, through our seventh chakra and our head, and then through the whole body all the way to our feet where the excess of energy goes into the Earth. When practicing this technique we continually let the energy flow through our body, and as a result our metabolism and metabolic processes speed up and our body cells are reinvigorated regularly. Furthermore, we also start feeling well and in harmony. Reiki teaches us to accept who we are and how we can find the optimal way of living a happy life within what was given to us when we were born. Reiki offers us life in accordance with the following affirmations: 'I am for a happy and harmonious life, I am for simplicity, I am for a direct communication with the outer world, I am for ....'

Naturally, Dr. Usui was not understood for many years and his technique was not accepted likewise. The simplicity of the idea and the absence of practitioner's dependence on the teacher were some of the main reasons why Reiki was not accepted as a self-healing technique. There are many stories about Dr. Usui's work and his attempts to share the Reiki technique with other people. Most of these stories are likely to be true and they all have one thing in common, and that is that he didn't live to see Reiki being accepted as an energy tool which can help people. In his lifetime, however, a story was going around about some excellent results of treatment conducted by means of this unresearched healing technique, and, due to that, Dr. Usui's family provided access to his papers after his death. After some years of research into his papers and into what Reiki was, his pupils and initiated masters Chujiro Hayashija and Hawayo Takate, a Hawaian, arranged the order of attunements into the Reiki symbols which were secretly being passed down from person to person for the following hundred years.

The secret passing of attunements was conditioned by the fact that both the followers and the students did not want to expose themselves to various inconveniences of being misunderstood as using some sort of 'magic'. So, the technique has been spreading slowly, but persistently, throughout the world until today when there are a few million people attuned into the Reiki symbols. Today Reiki is a popular self-healing technique which is accessible to everyone. There are visible healing results achieved by people who practice Reiki every day. The very technique is a simple and useful tool by means of which the outer energy is passed through the body which is then harmonized in its being. Two approaches to using symbols still prevail. One is the so-called traditional approach which is mysterious and tends to keep the names and forms of the symbols secret. The other is the modern approach which is open and without any secrets about how the symbols should be passed down. My experience from Tibet has taught me that Reiki is a natural technique and there is no need for shrouding it in secrecy. On one occasion, in one of Lhasa streets I met a Tibetan. After we had discussed the use and possibilities of this energy tool of placing palms on the body, this man showed me he didn't know what this tool was called, but despite that he was using it every day. Then I drew the first symbol in the sand, and he responded by drawing the second symbol, and then together we drew the third symbol, both of us smiling happily. After that, we met several times in the town and we always greeted each other by drawing the second symbol which in translation meant: 'I am happy to see you'. He always smiled happily and was overwhelmed by the fact that we managed to find a direct way of communicating without knowing each other's language.

There are two streams of Reiki teachers. The first are the so-called traditional teachers who are sensitive about groups of Reiki teachers being recognized, and who are full of mysterious information, starting from the fact that symbols should be kept secret and so on. The other teachers are the so-called modern teachers. They teach the Reiki technique which is based on enjoying the life without limitations and useless rituals which may only complicate the contact with the energy as well as create a feeling of insecurity about the correct way of using the energy. It is known that by imposing strict limitations on what is possible we are playing God, thus inhibiting both our personal and other people's growth. We all come from the Idea or God, so we are all perfect because God cannot create something imperfect. We are all unique and special at the same time, and as such we are welcome into being. Therefore, any potential limitations can only prevent people from growing and eventually result in boredom. Knowing people who persistently practice the traditional approach to Reiki, I have discovered that after they had practiced it for a few years, they stopped doing it as they simply got bored with repeating one and the same thing every day, and such approach couldn't bring them any closer to their inner selves. On the contrary, by introducing freedom to create your Reiki treatments and adapt them on the spot to suit the situation you are in, you are opening the way for exploring something new every day, and that is when the inner growth towards your inner self takes place.

It depends on your character and the energy of your master teacher if you are more for traditional or new and modern approach to Reiki. The choice of master is also an important step in adopting this simple and very efficient spiritual technique, which fills your physical, emotional and spiritual being with energy coming from the Universe. This energy comes in boundless quantities in the Universe, especially from the aspect of our individual life expectancy, so it is completely up to you to use it according to your needs. When you are spending time with Reiki you don't have to restrain yourself or be modest; just ask for as much as you need at that very moment. Any excess of energy will go through your feet into the Earth, thus feeding it as well.

As a supporter of the modern and playful approach to Reiki, I do not want to mention the name of my master teacher to whom I am tremendously grateful for moving me into this wonderful and flexible energy. I refuse mentioning her name not because I do not like her, but because I teach the participants of the course to be grateful only to the Universe, universal energies and their light guides who, in the most favorable way, lead them and guide them to use Reiki in their everyday life. Excessive gratitude is not needed as well as creating a strong bond between master-teacher and participant of the course, because all of us teachers are nothing more than transmitters-teachers showing this useful and simple tool to our students, and then it is up to them to use it. Constant gratitude to the teacher makes it impossible for the student to realize their self and to use Reiki only as a tool for collecting the requisite energy, while their personal awareness and talents should lead them on their light path so that they do not have to follow anyone, not even an enlightened person or a master-teacher of the Reiki technique. What a beauty when the student makes a step forward or anything more than their teacher, because at that very moment a growth in the structure of that person's consciousness takes place, and as a result another step in the growth of the vertical evolution happens, the evolution of consciousness!

This is where the idea for this book came from, because this book is meant to be an essential guide to possible uses of the Reiki symbols, and I kindly ask every person to add their own ideas about the ways in which they use the cosmic energy in their lives.

There is another important question that comes up at every course:

☉ Can the Reiki treatment and symbols solve all our problems?

I always respond in the same way:

☉ 'Yes, they can. They can solve all those problems which we truly want to solve. Because, if by doing the Reiki treatments I managed to free myself from colitis – inflammation of intestines, excess kilos and a series of complicated relationships, I do not see a reason why you couldn't do the same in your lives. We just have to make a decision and start using the energy carried by the symbols, but we should do this thoroughly and with our hearts open, with lots of love and understanding for ourselves, and the results will not fail to appear.'

A great problem which seems insuperable to a lot of people is the choice of the right master-teacher. The first and most important advice is not to expect from your master-teacher to be the person who will take on the responsibility for your being. They are here only to teach you the Reiki technique and to share with you their insights about you and your possibilities. After that, it is always up to you to choose where you will move on, at every crossroads of your being. Occasionally your master-teacher may show you what is behind each of the roads at a certain crossroads, but it is completely up to you to decide where to go by being fully responsible for all taken choices. If it was the contrary, the master-teacher would be playing God which would not do any good to both master-teacher and student. Also, if you stand in awe of your teacher, if you feel you cannot reach them and have confidence in them, then you are not on a good path; that is not your teacher. If, on the contrary, you feel comfortable, calm and pleased, and you feel understanding when meeting your master-teacher for the first time, it means that that person is the right master-teacher for you.

Chapter 4: What Is Reiki?

What is Reiki? Reiki is a Japanese form of Divine healing energy. In different cultures it may be called life force or Chi. Reiki is made up of 2 ancient Japanese kanji characters. The first one means "soul" or "spiritual." Ki, the second kanji symbol means "energy."

Reiki was developed by Master Mikao Usui who was said to have studies Buddhist sutras, martial arts, and other mystical arts. Master Usui fasted for 21 day and saw Reiki energy above his head. He developed Reiki and the symbols from this process and passed on the mysterious knowledge and symbols to several of his students. Some of the Reiki symbols used in healing are from Japanese Buddhism, Shinto and ancient Indian Sanskrit words.

Reiki is not a religion; it is a spiritual healing art that is from the Divine Source.

It is used to help the receiver, and the Reiki practitioner heal from the Reiki energy on spiritual, physical, emotional, and mental levels. Reiki can be done at a distance or directly with hands on the receiver. These methods are a catalyst to help one become healed, self-realized, enlightened, and have an open loving heart.

A Reiki practitioner has received attunements from one or more Reiki Masters. These initiations open up and connect the Reiki practitioner to the spiritual healing energy. Anyone can learn this ancient healing art. Anyone can receive this form of healing. It can help heal people, animals, and the earth. It doesn't go against any religion or spiritual practice.

The energy practitioner may lay their hands on the person receiving healing in a set structure of positions from the head, throat, chest, torso, legs and feet. The Reiki practitioner may stray away from these hand positions if they are guided to do so by their intuition or guides. Some Reiki practitioners may have their hands away from your body as well. Reiki may also be done from a distance, even across the globe! These methods can balance the chakras and subtle energy levels.

Practitioners learn the basic hand positions from a Reiki Master in Reiki I. The student then follows with a 21 day cleanse. This process has 12 hand positions that is done for one hour each day. This cleanse connects the new Reiki practitioner daily with this universal energy. It also helps the practitioner become more sensitive to subtle energies in and around their own body.

In Reiki II the student is introduced to the 3 basic, yet powerful symbols which intensify the Reiki energy. In Reiki II, the distance healing symbol is learned. In Reiki III More symbols are introduced. Reiki practitioners may take more classes, but some Masters allow one to teach after 3 classes. If you would like to learn more about Reiki, just ask!

REIKI PRINCIPLES

Reiki is the teaching of the Japanese holistic healing idea. There are a few differences between the Japanese and Western versions although it is really just a difference in the way things are done. One thing is that the Western version doesn't practice breathing techniques. With this practice you sit straight up in a chair and breathe in and out through the nose. At that time the energy enters through the top of the head.

Another difference between the two is the ways of treatment. In traditional Japanese healing people go to meetings every week and meditation work is done on separate parts, and with Western areas, the healing is usually done on the whole body. Also in Western areas there are three degrees or levels.

The first Reiki Degree course can be varied depending on the teacher. Some teachers have two classes over a two day period. Other teachers have four sessions spread over an extended period. Students are taught meditation and hand placement for healing. At that time they can heal themselves and others.

In the second degree level students learn the use of symbols to enhance the connection between the healer and recipient. The use of these symbols helps to do the healing over distance and time. You can heal people without being with them. In Japan it has been known to take ten to twenty years to attain the second degree. It is dependent on the teacher.

In Reiki, there is always learning involved. As with the third degree, there is a time that it takes to study and practice. It depends on the teacher as to how long it takes to attain third degree status. It could be a day or a year or more. When you are obtaining the third degree you are given another symbol.

It is thought that Reiki healing is used on the front and back of the body equally. It is usually started at the head and neck and then the other parts of the body. Reiki does not use medicine or instruments but feeling, blowing, tapping, and massaging. It is a practice that uses the energies that surround all of us always.

Many Western practitioners usually use a standard twelve positions for whole body healing. The recipient is asked to lay down when this is being done. The hands are usually held at each position for five minutes. Some people say that they get a warm feeling where the treatment is being applied. This is also a hand off treatment as the hands are held as few centimeters away from the recipient.

There is really no governing board for Reiki practitioners but there are organizations that want to standardize Reiki practices. If that should happen the practice might be under government regulation and that could be a fatal blow the practitioners of today and of the future.

WHAT IS REIKI INITIATION AND HOW CAN IT HELP YOU

Reiki, as is well-known, is a derivation of Buddhist philosophies, which a Buddhist monk name Masai Ukui derived in Japan during a spiritual retreat in the 19th century. Reiki has become massively popular in Western culture due to the claims made on its behalf - it is stated by reiki teachers and master that reiki can help ease a sufferer's pain while supplementing his or her regular medical treatment.

This is something to remember: reiki is not a replacement for mainstream modern medicine. Buddhist philosophy explicitly states that it is designed for the easing of a person's pain, and reiki itself is derived from such teachings. Reiki works on spiritual energies, which are contained in the body of the sufferer and, if misaligned, cause pain. These energy or 'ki' sites are the basis of reiki practice, and there are three levels of proficiency. Let's take a quick look at each.

During a reiki course the student undergoes a process of attunement, or initiation, under the tutelage of a Reiki master. Very simply, this allows the student to use and receive more of the universal spiritual energy circulating around us. The rate at which this energy spins differs, and so there must be different techniques and methods of dealing with it.

These methods are taught at the ascending levels of reiki studenthood, at the final stage of which one is considered a reiki master. These levels are Reiki 1, Reiki 2, and the third, Level 3, at which one is considered a master and can go forth and train more budding recruits into the ranks of the reiki elite. It is possible, with the recent advances made in the teaching of reiki, to advance to the second level in a matter of mere days.

The attunement process starts with the master reflecting this universal energy, via his or her hands, into the body of the sufferer. The person's body is then searched for hidden blockages of the energy, the 'ki', which is the basis of every human being's spiritual self.

In order, the process goes through the following three stages:

The Reiki initiation level 1 works by stimulating the body to receive a small amount of spiritual energy, and to prepare it to receive more. This is a complete novice level. It also makes the person who receives this initiation capable of retaining that attunement for the rest of his or her life. The basic hand positions of reiki, as well as some of its history, are taught, and at the end of each experience - always relaxing and spiritually good for both master and student - the student can progress to the second level, or choose to remain at level 1 and continue to experience the good it does to him or her.

The Reiki initiation level 2 involves the teaching of certain symbols, e.g. the mental symbol, which then allow the student to prepare for the third level, which is where the student achieves mastery.

THINGS YOU NEED WHEN STARTING YOUR REIKI PRACTICE

Are you a trained in Reiki and want to start making a living of it? Are you setting up your own Reiki practice? Congratulations! You are going to make a difference in many people's lives. So what do you need when starting out, apart from the legalities and a location to practice? In this article I will go through the equipment that you will need and I hope it will prove useful information.

1. Reiki Table. This can mean an important investment as some of them don't come very cheap. But don't just look at the price. You need to see the whole picture. A high quality table, with a long warranty, will pay you its cost many times over. You need to make sure the measures are adequate and that it is portable. Make sure it is sturdy and that it feels stable. Your clients won't feel secure when lying down otherwise. The Reiki tables differ from normal massage tables in one aspect. Reiki tables have room for your legs so that you can sit next to it comfortably. Massage tables usually don't have this feature because the therapist spends more time standing then sitting down.

2. Reiki Table Carrying case. Some sellers will include a carrying case in the package, and if not I very much recommend getting one separately. Maybe you have clients that are too ill to get to your practice and you need to do a lot of home visits. This can easily be arranged if your equipment is

light and portable. A carrying case can be useful even if you don't move about a lot, when storing it for example.

3. Reiki Table accessories. This is up to every Reiki practitioner but the basics are usually face and head rest, adjustable arm rest and bolster.

4. Clean linens, preferably white. There are special ones made for massage and Reiki tables that fit perfectly.

5. Blankets and pillows to assure maximum comfort. Choose natural materials such as cotton, not synthetics.

6. Decoration. This is very subjective. Some Reiki practitioners will decorate the room with crystals, posters, candles. This is really up to each and every one of us but make sure you choose only authentic products. You should feel a positive energy when walking into the practice, and so should your clients.

7. Relaxing music and stereo equipment.

8. Crystals. Some Reiki experts say that crystals used during Reiki will help the healing and energy balancing. And they also speed up the recovery process. You can start with a small collection of stones. They shouldn't be too heavy nor too small that you'll lose them. Flat stones will stay on the spot more easily. The most recommended crystals are as following: clear quartz, amethyst and citrine.

Chapter 5: What Is Reiki?

What comes to your mind when you see or hear the word Reiki? Does it remind you of an herbal tea brand? Do you envision those luscious landscapes in paintings? Do you think of it as ancient symbols? Whatever came to your thoughts, Reiki is not any of them. In truth, it means a lot more than you think.

Definition

The word "Reiki", which comes from the Japanese words 'rei' (universal) and 'ki' (life energy), means "mysterious atmosphere, miraculous sign." It also denotes "spiritually guided life energy." As you may have guessed, Reiki is a type of energy healing. It helps heal a person through the energy fields around their body. Reiki can also be seen as a technique to reduce stress and promote relaxation.

What many are not aware of is that Reiki is a foundation of three methods derived from Japan: Kenyoku Ho, Joshin Kokyu Ho, and Seishin Toitsu. They encourage spiritual work, energy cleansing, and breathing exercises, which Reiki is all about.

Reiki takes place through various techniques where the hands are positioned to feel the energy fields around one's body. This is where the practitioner can feel how life energy flows and administer the healing process to help the patient let go of stress, pain, anxiety, and other negative things from within.

Also, when one wishes to learn how to use Reiki, it is not taught like most healing practices. The ability is actually passed on from the master to the student during an attunement. This means that the student has access to a limitless supply of energy that can help them improve their health, detoxify their bodies, and heal others.

Reiki is not tied to any specific religion, so it is available to everyone and can be taught to millions of people from all walks of life. Because of its spiritual nature, Reiki can be used by both believers and non-believers. It also helps them become religious since Reiki is supposed to come from God.

Reiki also encourages everyone to live in peace and harmony while being respectful and courteous with others.

Worldwide Reception

Though Reiki has gained praise because of its benefits, methods, and reviews, its reception worldwide is a mixed bag. Many experts classify Reiki healing as a pseudoscience because its authenticity doesn't have strong scientific evidence. There are even articles claiming that the benefits of Reiki need to be further researched. Others have also conducted studies of their own to prove that the practice has several shortcomings. It has been seen as a concern for the Catholic church in the past as well. Then, some people insist that Reiki is bad, so they have been writing flaming articles to bring its reputation down.

Others have also complained about Reiki healing being a scam. When you check out the pricing and offers that the practitioners have, you can see that the cost can be a bit high. In truth, there was a time when Reiki healing cost about $10000 per session. This has given its reception a bad vibe and has caused many folks to wonder if it is even worth spending money on.

Despite all that, the individuals who have experienced healing through Reiki have fought back and tried to prove the naysayers wrong, giving examples of why its benefits are real. Reiki has been proven to be advantageous in other areas, such as sports, alternative healing methods, wellness routines, and many more. Many have compiled testimonials from people who have tried the practice and shared how their pain, suffering, and other negativities they once had were all banished. Some of them have even become licensed practitioners themselves and put their knowledge into good use after ascending the levels and going through the attunements. You can search about them through Google and get started with a healing session right away if you want.

Whichever opinion you stand for, one thing is for certain: Reiki is here to stay, and it will continue to grow as more and more people learn and master the art of channeling universal energy and using it for healing purposes.

Chapter 6: Understanding Reiki

There is a common misconception that Reiki is the belief in a higher power. Yet you do not have to change your belief system in order to practice or benefit from Reiki. The origin of this practice is not quite known, but during the 1920's, a Japanese man by the name of Usui Sensei rediscovered the art of Reiki. On a pilgrimage to a waterfall known for meditation purposes, Kurama Yama, Usui Sensei fasted for twenty-one days before he discovered the Reiki practice. When he came back from his fast, he told his family of having been struck through the top of the head with a strong power, and how that power had taught him how to use the power within him to heal others.

Western Reiki is somewhat different from the traditional Japanese Reiki because the woman who introduced it to Western society, Hawayo Takata, tweaked it in order for it to be more acceptable to Western society's standards. Mrs. Takata learned from Hayashi Sensei, the successor of the original Reiki Master, Usui Sensei. Her story goes like this:

Mrs. Takata's sister died, which required her to travel to Japan to tell her parents about her sister's death. At the time, she was suffering from abdominal and lung pain which were caused by a tumor, gallstones, appendicitis, and asthma. She believed she could receive treatment for these ailments in Japan and went to a hospital where she was diagnosed. She had heard about Reiki and wanted to try that before she underwent extensive surgery to cure her.

Mrs. Takata began Reiki treatment under the supervision of Hayashi Sensei. She received treatment twice daily from two practitioners and the heat from their hands was so great that she thought they were treating her with a device hidden in their sleeves. And so she decided to grab the sleeve of one practitioner to see if he indeed had a device up there, but she found nothing. That was when the practitioners gladly told her how Reiki worked. Fascinated, she continued to receive treatment for four months and was eventually cured of her ailments.

Mrs. Takata teamed up with Hayashi Sensei in order to figure out how they could bring this wonderful practice to the West. In the year, 1937, she went back to Hawaii accompanied by Hayashi Sensei and his daughter. There, they set up a Reiki facility, and in 1938, she was initiated as Reiki Master. From then on, she spread the practice of Reiki to her students and they spread their knowledge to others. Reiki has become a worldwide practice due to Mrs. Takata's persistence.

While most people who practice Reiki have some sort of belief in a higher power, it is more about being a spiritual being. Just believing that we have energy flowing through our bodies that is capable of healing ourselves and our fellow men is enough to begin implementing the practice of Reiki. Reiki, as a word, actually carries the meaning of spiritually guided life force energy.

This form of treatment for all manner of physical; mental; and even emotional maladies works by creating a feeling of relaxation, peace, security, and well-being. Its purpose is to help people understand that they can heal their bodies and spirits consciously. In order for this form of healing to work, the patient must understand that they are taking just as much responsibility for their healing as the person helping them. This might be easier to do if you are the one performing the ritual on yourself, something which is commonly practiced amongst many Reiki students and teachers. After all, how can we understand what we are doing if we are not trying it on ourselves?

So what is it, exactly?

Reiki is using the energy within you, a healing energy, and projecting it to create balance in the human energy fields, or auras and chakras in order to create the conditions that are needed for our bodies to function properly when healing. The energy is transmitted through our hands and realigns the energy of the other person or ourselves, in order for our bodies to heal. It can be used for any ailment of the body, mind, or psyche.

Some of the more common health benefits Reiki patients and practitioners report are:

A deep relaxation that helps the person relax and release stress and tension

An acceleration in the body's healing abilities

Better sleep

Reduction in blood pressure

Acute injuries and chronic problems, including addiction, are healed

Relief of pain

Readjustment of the energy in the endocrine system which allows the body to heal

Assists in cleaning toxins

Helps the body heal after drug therapies used after surgery and chemotherapy

Boosts the immune system

Increases vitality

Helps in clearing your emotions and growing spiritually

There are numerous reasons why people use Reiki, but the main goal of the practice is to help the human body and spirit to heal.

To better understand Reiki, it is best to understand the human chakras and auras, which are discussed in the following chapter.

Chapter 7: Reiki Symbols

There are typically five traditional symbols in Reiki that help enhance the depth of connectivity between the practitioner and the universal energy. It is important to remember that the symbols by themselves have little or no influence on the healing. The strength and intention of the symbol are directly dependent on the meditative and intentional powers of the practitioner.

The Power Symbol

The Power Symbol is called Cho Ku Rei and is shaped like a coil. This coil-shaped Reiki symbol can be drawn clockwise or counter-clockwise to increase positive energy or decrease negative energy respectively. The Cho Ku Rei facilitates the practitioner in regulating the universal energy referred to as Qi or Ki.

The clockwise direction of the coil creates an expansion of energy and the counter-clockwise direction results in energy contract. Depending on the Reiki need, the practitioner chooses to draw the Power Symbol in the required direction. The Cho Ku Rei also provides emotional, mental, and physical protection to the practitioner and the Reiki receiver.

The Harmony Symbol

Referred to as Sei Hei Ki, the Harmony Symbol in Reiki resembles the expanded wings of a bird in flight or a wave washing ashore. The Harmony Symbol is drawn with a sweeping gesture. The purpose of this symbol is purification and is used frequently by practitioners for emotional and mental healing.

The Harmony Symbol is typically used to help people overcome addictions and depression by helping to restore the spiritual equilibrium. The Harmony Symbol is also used to overcome the pains and agonies of past, unresolved traumas and to remove energy blockages. It is very effective for healing deep-rooted emotional traumas.

The Distance Symbol

Referred to as Hon Sha Ze Sho Nen, the Distance Symbol, as the name suggests, is used to send Ki during remote Reiki sessions to people located at a long distance from the practitioner. When the characters of the Distance Symbol are written down, it looks like a tower, and therefore, is also called pagoda. The intention of this symbol is to bring together people across space and time.

Another unique power of this symbol is that it can be converted to form a key that opens the Akashi records believed to be the source of all human consciousness. Practitioners use the power and intention of this symbol to deal with past-life and inner-child experiences of clients.

The Distance Symbol can also be used in cases where a situation calls for the healer not to touch the client for some reason.

The Master Symbol

The Master Symbol, called Dai Ko Myo, stands for all that is Reiki. The purpose of the Master Symbol is enlightenment. It is a complex symbol to draw, and Reiki Masters use only this for attunements. The Master Symbol combines the power of distance, harmony, and power symbols to heal the healers.

The Completion Symbol

Referred to as Raku symbol, the Completion Symbol that looks like a striking bolt of lightning is used in the last stages of the attunement process. The intention of the Completion is 'grounding.' As the name suggests, the Completion Symbol is used to settle the body and mind and seal the awakened Ki after the attunement is completed. The practitioner draws this symbol by hand in the downward direction reflecting the completion of the attunement process.

Typically, these symbols can be used only by those who have been attuned to the second level of Reiki.

Chapter 8: The Sensation Of Reiki

If you have read the first part of this book "The Healing Power of Reiki", it is clear that you have been introduced to what Reiki is capable of doing for one's health. It is not a practice that has empirical evidence to suggest that it can cure just about any diseases. But for those who have "felt" the touch of Reiki in their lives, they can safely say that it has transformed them.

Now, what does invisible but powerful energy feel like? When a person performs or receives Reiki, what are the sensations that go on in the body? Here is a brief understanding of the sensation of Reiki.

The Movement of Reiki

Reiki is energy and energy flows from one person to the next. Now, the first thing that you will notice with Reiki is that it works almost like a thermostat for the body. The flow of Reiki can either be fast or slow depending upon how the balancing energies are dispensed. It swings back and forth, sometimes erratically and sometimes very smoothly. When the energy fluctuates within the body, different people describe it differently. Some say that it feels like you are experiencing hot flashes, throbbing pulses all over the body, chills, pin pricks or a mild sensation of tingling.

During a Reiki session, it is not just the receiver but also the practitioner who feels several sensations. The first sensation experienced by the practitioners is the heating up of his palms. This is because the energy is being transmitted from the palm to the body of the receiver. The receiver, on the other hand, is able to feel the body relaxing completely. They tend to yawn a lot during the session because the body begins to let go of all the stress. Unless you are in good tune with your body, it is very difficult to explain these sensations very specifically, especially if you are on the receiving end of the Reiki session.

No sensations at all

If you speak to people who have had any experience of Reiki in their lives, they will tell you that they have heard certain inner voices, have seen very vivid images and have even felt extreme fluctuations in temperatures. Now, if you are someone who has felt absolutely nothing during your Reiki session or practice, do not panic. It does not mean that Reiki is not working for you. It only means that you need to focus a little more. Try to receive your Reiki session in a room that has no visual distraction so that your focus is entirely on the reception of energy.

What do hot hands mean?

When individuals get a Reiki attunement, they begin to believe that they need to develop hot hands. Yes, it is true that when an individual becomes a channel for

Reiki energy, it awakens in the form of heat on your palm. While this may indicate that your Reiki energy is functioning, it is not the only indication of attunement. If someone tells you that your experience of Reiki was insufficient because of a lack of heat formation, do not be misled by it.

Temperature may vary

In case of a few practitioners of Reiki, the temperature of the hand keeps changing as the treatment continues. Sometimes it is very hot and other times it is as cold as ice. There are also variations in the way people perceive the temperatures. The receiver may feel like the hands of the practitioner are cold while the practitioner might be experiencing a burning sensation on the palm of his hands.

Extra hands for healing

Sometimes, you may feel like there are other practitioners in the room who are participating in the session with you. These hands will feel like they have been placed on your body. This is a very common sensation in Reiki, although it may seem a little strange at first. Now, according to Maureen J. Kelly who is the author of the Healing Buddha, the extra hands could be the result of other healing spirit guides that are present in the room with you.

The Pulse of Reiki

There are several people who feel a tingling, pulsating sensation all over their body. This sensation, however, is not felt on the hands. The palm is the channel from which the Reiki energy leaves you and moves out. When you have been attuned you will constantly feel this Reiki energy wanting to break out of your body and move right out of your palms. That is why you feel the pulsating sensation. So the moment you place your hand on the body of another person, you will feel the energy come alive automatically.

Many Reiki practitioners describe themselves as a live generator. The body heats up and begins to generate the energy out to anyone who is even slightly receptive to this energy. Sometimes, people who have just received their attunement, they can wrongly believe that the person who is open to the Reiki sensation needs it. Do not touch the other person or perform any Reiki on them without receiving their permission first. This is a rule that you need to follow. What you need to understand is that the pulsating sensation is so strong that you may not really think about what you are doing.

There are other times when you feel like the energy of Reiki is forming a ball on your palm. It is almost like you have a tennis ball on your palm. Now, you cannot shake this energy off as this is being generated from you and is as alive as you are. Initially, this may seem a little uncomfortable and will make you feel like the energy is almost getting drained from you. That, however, is not true. Unless you have someone who can receive your Reiki energy it will not leave your palm. This balling up of energy on your palm is an indication that you may be in the need for self Reiki. So just place your hands on your body when you feel this energy and release the tension that you are feeling in your hands.

Transferring the energy

As you practice Reiki, the energy will only get stronger. Sometimes, you are physically able to experience this energy building up within your body. Many practitioners who are able will actually transfer this energy to inanimate objects to just get it out of their own system. It is possible to transfer your excess energy into another object when you just place it between your palms. Here are a few options for transferring your Reiki energy.

You may place the energy inside your pillow case to make sure that you get better sleep, it can be transferred into water to make the water more refreshing, it can even be transferred into your toothpaste, lotions and shampoos to improve their effect.

Vibrations and other sensations

As the Reiki energy is being transferred around your body, it makes adjustments to flow easily through your body. This may lead to vibrations that you will feel very strongly on the palms of your hands. This is because the energy that is gushing around the body almost stops at your palm when it is not being transferred. It feels like the energy is actually struggling to get out.

There are other Reiki sensations such as mild pain in the joints of the finger and the wrists. When you are treating severe problems or illnesses, you can even feel this soreness on your back, shoulders and neck. For those who find this type of energy transfer painful or uncomfortable, it is recommended that you take your hands off, rest them and then proceed again.

What you need to understand with Reiki energy is that it will make its own path of flow. That is why each person's experience with it is so different and unique. Never be afraid of the Reiki sensations. Instead, find ways to master the energy and control its effect.

Chapter 9: Why Offer Reiki To Cats?

Animals that live in close connection with humans become their companions and confidants, providing them with comfort protection, and unconditional love. This relationship often results in the internalization of their human companion's problems and stress, which can later be manifested as undesired physical and mental behaviors in the animals.

Reiki energy is beneficial for animals because it is safe, non-invasive, and gentle in nature. It facilitates the animal's ability to heal itself naturally and complements all other forms of healing treatments. Reiki energy, however, is not a substitute for the need to consult with a veterinary professional regarding both urgent and on-going medical care for your animal companions.

- Reiki energy accelerates the healing of physical injury or illness and facilitates the treatment of behavioral problems that may surface due to emotional issues with an animal.

- Reiki energy induces deep relaxation, assists in the reduction of stress, and promotes feelings of calm, trust, safety, and peace in animals.

- Reiki treatments may be hands-on or they may be offered to an animal from any distance away with the same level of intensity and effect.

- Reiki creates a special connection between the practitioner and the animal, which allows the animal to become an active participant in its own healing process instead of merely being a passive recipient of the treatment.

- Reiki can do no harm and always heals on some level – even if changes in the animal's condition or behavior are not immediately apparent.

· Reiki can help to ease the transition from life to death for both animal and human by providing relief from fear, anxiety, and pain.

The ability to channel Reiki energy to animals can be easily learned from a qualified Reiki Master-Teacher by animal owners, as well as by veterinarians, groomers, trainers, therapists, and shelter/rescue staff and volunteers. Animals themselves may be attuned to Reiki energy to become Animal Reiki Healers.

Since animals are much more sensitive to their health and energy than humans are, they tend to feel Reiki energy very easily and quickly. An animal's reaction to Reiki will vary based on its temperament and prior experiences with humans – ranging from quick and eager acceptance to outright and even aggressive rejection of the energy. When they are open to the energy, animals will often guide attention to areas of their bodies that are most in need of healing.

Chapter 10: The Importance Of Initiation Size

Reiki is an approach to utilize the vitality in your grasp to adjust and revive the existence power vitality inside us. At the point when our life power vitality is high, we are less inclined to become ill. Numerous individuals who have been sick have profited by physical, mental and passionate recuperating from this hands-on vitality treatment. Through Reiki attunements, you can figure out how to take advantage of the existence power vitality and renew and mend yourself as well as other people. For some, the attunement or commencement procedure begins in 1stDegree Reiki Practitioners Healing Training. For other people, it is the formal commencement into mending others performed at the Reiki ace level.

This book examines the job of attunement in Levels 1, 2 and Masters Reiki preparing.

With numerous reports in the media about vitality mending, more individuals are interested and looking for an introduction to vitality recuperating. Standard Reiki attunements is a demonstrated method to guarantee long haul great health. One of the attractions of Reiki is that anybody can figure out how to utilize it. Reiki bosses mend by widespread vitality, or Qi, that is gone through the palms. This life renewing vitality practice is passed on from ace to student.

Reiki doesn't just treat physical wellbeing yet in addition enthusiastic, mental and otherworldly health. Ensuring your life power vitality is adjusted is the most ideal approach to guarantee all encompassing wellbeing. This Japanese recuperating strategy is progressively being utilized close by Western prescription as a component of the mending process. Thus, request is expanding for prepared experts who can perform Reiki attunements.

Solution to choosing Reiki Initiation Master

Picking the privilege Reiki ace is essential to the achievement of your attunements in every one of the three degrees of training. Since Mikao Usui created Reiki in 1922, numerous varieties have pursued. Request that your planned educator clarify their preparation and experience utilizing Reiki. Ask her to discuss her way of thinking of Reiki and bow it might contrast from that of other Reiki masters. And critically, get some information about any progressions or upgrades to her Reiki program from the customary practice.

The International Center for Reiki, for instance, underlines the convention of the customary Tibetan methods just as the Usui Reiki techniques. This program professes to make changes in accordance with the first Reiki technique. truth be told, there are a few ancestries of Reiki instructed in Japan today – some of them hidden and others vigorously impacted by the Western procedures. Guarantee you comprehend the Reiki procedure being offered. Specifically inquire as to why this framework is the best for you.

Functional contemplations incorporate booking. When is the class held and for how long? Weekend courses have turned out to be well known however would a weeklong retreat be better for you? Charges shift extraordinarily today among schools. To direct Reiki to other people, every one of the three levels are required. At the ace level, you will be started into recuperating others. Consider at the time, cash and different assets you will require to finish Masters level Reiki.

Reiki is more physically private than many specialist understanding relationships. Ask yourself how agreeable you would lie on a table for an hour getting Reiki medications from your educator. Reiki includes opening yourself up profoundly and emotionally. If you wind up inclination guarded or bashful, keep on talking Reiki teachers. Assess your mood. Do feel upbeat around this person? Does the educator make you like yourself?

Planning for the Attunement Process

Clear your calendar of all commitments. If you have a ton of work and family worry during your Reiki class, it will be more earnestly to open yourself up to the vitality procedure. Try not to design any significant get-togethers during your Reiki commencement forms, particularly those including liquor.

Sanitize your arrangement of poisons. Take out caffeine, liquor, meat and sugar from your diet. Consider fasting for a couple of days.

Think for an hour every day. This is a significant advance that will enable you to quiet your psyche and manage your vitality stream before the exercises start. You will get more from Reiki preparing Assuming you are now raising your vitality vibrations.

Attempt and maintain a strategic distance from unpleasant circumstances and individuals. Once more, this is to help guarantee a quiet, thoughtful attitude.

Invest more energy among nature. Another unwinding strategy. Stroll to take a shot at a bright day. Take a walk around the recreation center or by the sea as opposed to staring at the TV.

The Reiki Attunement Process

What is Reiki Initiation?

Ace Usui got his capacity to take advantage of Reiki vitality through an otherworldly reflection. The custom of passing Reiki down from ace to understudy proceeds. Attunement is another and later term for Initiation, or reiju in Japanese. Pamela Miles, a Reiki specialist, makes a noteworthy distinction between the terms attunement and inception in her blog. Understanding the genuine significance of inception will extend your Reiki practice. Quickly, attunement is frequently characterized as the strict exchange of all inclusive vitality from ace to understudy, supplying the understudy with the capacity to turn into a healer. Though inception alludes to the start of learning a training. Learning, as Miles notes, includes posing inquiries, and learning can be constant. Like the nonstop renewal of vitality, the professional ought to constantly build up their abilities as a vitality healer. While inception better catches the genuine plan of Reiki recuperating, we will keep on utilizing the famous term attunement here. Yet rather than consider attunement a privilege of entry as a vitality healer, attempt and think about every attunement procedure as the start of a constant learning process.

Reiki Attunement : An approach Through the Three Reiki Levels

The attunement or commencement procedure happens in every one of the three degrees of Reiki: Reiki 1, Reiki 2, and Master level. At each level the Master starts the understudy with more grounded mending vitality as the understudy moves to more elevated amounts of vitality vibration.

Reiki 1 includes four commencements of the physical body. To become an affirmed level 1 Reiki expert, you will find out about the vitality meridians of the body, the Reiki hand positions, and Reiki life systems; and at last how to utilize the Reiki vitality framework to recuperate yourself as well as other people. When this learning is effectively aced, the Level 1 Reiki attunement must be given by a Certified Reiki Master. The function more often than not takes 20 or 30 minutes.

Reiki 2 starts the unpretentious or air body. Three Reiki images are educated – control, mental and separation. Notwithstanding the sacrosanct symbols, 2ndDegree Certified Reiki Practitioners Training teaches extra images and hand positions. A few courses will likewise show removed Reiki recuperating at this stage.

The Reiki Master level starts the understudy into instructing Reiki. The Master image is educated. A few Masters allude to this third organize as the official attunement or inception arrange as a vitality healer. At Level 3, you will figure out how to do Reiki attunement on others.

Separation Reiki Attunement

Numerous individuals offer the chance to get Reiki and different types of vitality mending a good ways off. While some separation healers have demonstrated that they draw from an amazing vitality source, most Reiki experts don't prescribe separation mending. Episodically, many people from those utilizing separation recuperating report that the vitality isn't as solid. A few bosses accept that the physical touch is basic to convey the required mending vitality. Handy contemplations incorporate challenges getting neighborhood references and joining nearby Reiki gatherings to whom your healer likewise has a place. In the case of preparing in Reiki or looking for mending, similar capabilities for picking a Reiki ace ought to be utilized.

The Reiki Ideals

Learning the Reiki procedures and going through all phases of attunement/inception is just piece of the way toward turning into a mindful vitality healer. You should likewise maintain the good and moral norms of a Reiki vitality healer. The Reiki Ideals were created by Reiki organizer Usui Mikao. The Reiki Ideals guarantee the sound and dependable routine with regards to Reiki. They are an attestation that you are the healer and in charge of your own demonstrations of mending. The first Reiki beliefs are as per the following:

· The mystery specialty of welcoming bliss

· The marvelous medication everything being equal

· Only for now, don't outrage

· Try not to stress and be loaded up with appreciation

· Dedicate yourself to your work. Be thoughtful to individuals.

· Each morning and night, join your hands in petition.

· Ask these words to your heart

· furthermore, serenade these words with your mouth

Check out Usui Reiki Treatment for the improvement of body and psyche

When you have learned Reiki, the capacity to mend yourself as well as other people physically, rationally, sincerely and profoundly is with you for a lifetime. Like any learning, Assuming you seek after nonstop learning – that is, continually addressing and finding out more – your Reiki mending vitality will stay solid and all the more profoundly receptive to the general vitality source. While recuperating others is a steady wellspring of reconnection with the vitality source, getting attunements now and again from different bosses will keep you finely sensitive to the vitality source.

Inception or attunement?

Some time after the demise of Hawayo Takata* in December 1980, "attunement" firing springing up. Numerous Reiki experts presently use it only for the procedure Mrs. Takata alluded to as inception (reiju in Japanese).

Be sure that the inception procedure is baffling, "commencement" is entirely clear. It alludes to starting.

Inception is the procedure by which an ace offers with an understudy the capacity to rehearse. Commencement ancestry keeps a training alive, and is regular in Asian profound customs.

The procedure of inception is innately baffling; what it achieves — empowering us to rehearse — isn't.

Similarly as the pith of training is to start once more, commencement can be rehashed. Usui offered reiju to his students each time they assembled to rehearse.

The ascent of "attunement" appears to have put a conclusion to addressing. It urged specialists to see Reiki as a specific vibration of "vitality" to which individuals should be "adjusted" so as to rehearse. This disarray — that one is receptive to vitality as opposed to started into training — has taken on its very own existence and is currently for the most part introduced as certainty.

In any case, it is anything but a reality. It's a conviction. What's more, if Reiki practice is predicated on conviction, it's never again a training; it turns into a religion.

When you notices it that way — which is how individuals outside the New Age people group will in general notices it — is it so astonishing that some religious society are against Reiki practice?

Demystifying inception, in a manner of speaking

It's difficult to really demystify inception in light of this fact, the procedure itself is supernatural. In any case, while the inception procedure is baffling, what it achieves is down to earth and normally unmistakable. Individuals who get a Reiki inception might possibly see something during the procedure of commencement, however I would say, they see the impact.

As a youthful Reiki ace, I committed the error maybe all new aces make: I blabbered.

After some time I came to welcome that my activity isn't to clarify Reiki. Or maybe, my duty as a Reiki ace is just to show understudies how to rehearse Reiki, to move them to rehearse day by day self-treatment, and to give them the certainty that they really can rehearse effectively.

Is inception enough?

I realize every one of my understudies need are the inceptions; I likewise realize they don't have the foggiest idea about that. I can't anticipate that them should trust me, nor do I need them to. I need understudies to build up their very own certainty. What's more, nothing I state can make certainty the path in-class practice does.

In my First degree classes, we move into the first of four inceptions offered in Hawayo Takata's genealogy directly after the welcome and presentations. I at that point lead the understudies through their first altered Reiki self practice. After this short introductory practice, and before they open their eyes, I request that they see any little contrast between the manner in which they feel currently contrasted with how they felt when they began.

When I've delicately driven them out of their training session, the understudies share what they saw during their first practice. I don't recall the last time somebody didn't see anything.

In any event, individuals feel more settled, increasingly focused, progressively loose — and that is not how they expected to feel sitting discreetly in a gathering of outsiders.

The procedure of commencement is innately secretive; what it achieves — empowering us to rehearse — isn't.

Reiki Initiations are here to push you to reconnect with your picked life way and to turn into a channel for this Universal Life Healing Energy. It is the establishment for your own healing in your consistently life and a chance to pass it onto other living creatures in the hour of this major vivacious progress from the third dimensional Energy to the fifth dimensional Energy. It is a mending practice and a method for living with profound regard, sympathy and empathy for the Soul and each living being including yourself, other individuals, creatures, plants and Mother Earth.

Reiki Initiations can raise your cognizance to a more prominent level and bring understanding of your actual way and subsequently the motivation to your own picked educational experience, the significance (or certainty) of disease or a problem, and learning involved. Through Reiki Initiations your own vitality is being raised, your levels of awareness and mindfulness start developing – so significant as of now of transformation, to stay aware of this approaching high fifth dimensional Energy.

SO DO WE NEED INITIATION TO BE ABLE TO USE REIKI?

Indeed, we should be started by a Reiki Master Teacher, who has been adjusted accurately themselves. Reiki is a high, sacred Life Healing Energy and to have the option to arrive at that level our energy and awareness should be raised. We can not do this by itself, a Reiki Master should be there for us to take us however those stages. This is the way Master Usui started his understudies. It is a significant minute in each person't life when we believe we are reconnecting with our actual self and the Holy Source that individuals call Mother/Father God.

In contrast to other recuperating expressions, Reiki is passed from ace to understudy through a Reiki attunement that allows the understudy to interface with the all inclusive Reiki source.

So, what is Involved for Each Reiki Attunement?

Be aware that in a Reiki level 1 attunement, students are receptive to three unique images, each speaking to an alternate part of Reiki vitality: control, mental/passionate equalization and separation recuperating. Every understudy gets attunements to these 3 images four separate occasions, and with every reiteration the association develops.

Therefore, the attunements for Reiki level 2 and Reiki ace are comparative in nature, yet include various images, each with an alternate importance to opening your vivacious pathways.

What feeling comes through Attunement?

Be aware that getting a Reiki attunement is a ground-breaking profound experience, as your lively pathways are opened by a Reiki ace. This vivacious opening permits the Reiki vitality to stream uninhibitedly through your body to affect your wellbeing and the soundness of others.

The sentiment of a Reiki attunement is an individual one, yet understudies regularly report that they feel a helping of their body and shivering from their head to their toes as the Reiki vitality pathways are opened.

The opening of an attunement has the impact of enhancing other lively mending and directing pathways, and understudies report that accepting an attunement causes expanded instinctive mindfulness, and improves any intrinsic clairvoyant affectability.

How Do You Prepare for an Attunement?

Meanwhile, how you get ready for a Reiki attunement relies upon your very own profound practice. Opening a vigorous pathway is no light issue, and keeping in mind that it's not carefully important to do anything so as to get ready to get a Reiki attunement, most understudies decide to reconnect with their own otherworldly practice before their attunement, to increase the general impacts of the attunement and amplify its transformative power.

One prescribed arrangement for planning for a Reiki attunement involves a 3-day rinse before your attunement. Abstain from eating overwhelming nourishments, limit or dispose of caffeine, sugar, tobacco or liquor. Invest your energy perusing or pondering instead of sitting in front of the TV. Endeavor to discharge negative feelings, for example, outrage or desire.

These arrangements will enable you to be increasingly prepared to acknowledge the otherworldly change and urge the attunement to have significant, long haul impacts on your life and prosperity.

Does an Attunement Need to be Renewed?

When you have been sensitive to Reiki, the Reiki vitality will course through you for an incredible remainder. Your capacity to channel and move Reiki vitality stays with you, as the endowment of Reiki tails you and encourages you for an incredible remainder.

So what Are the Benefits of Receiving Attunements Remotely?

In-person classes are regularly instructed rapidly, absent much time for understudies to consolidate the data. The attunements are given as once huge mob toward the part of the arrangement, without time for the understudies to plan for the significant otherworldly change that an attunement involves. By studying remotely, you can learn and incorporate the advantages of Reiki at your own pace, and take a couple of days to set yourself up for your attunement before you get it.

Reiki is an enthusiastic practice, and a great part of the Reiki you get and convey all through a mind-blowing remainder will be a ways off. Starting your Reiki venture remotely encourages you get ready for an existence of Reiki without outskirts.

Chapter 11: The Principles Of Reiki

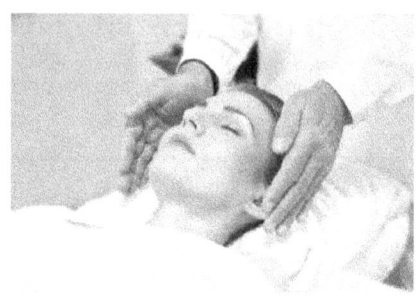

Reiki has five principles that govern it. These principles bring fulfillment to anyone who lives according to them. The principles will a lot of value in your life and bring you the balance you did not have. Anyone is not restricted to live obeying theses spiritual ideals, but once you decide to learn and live by the principles, you will find yourself liking them and putting them to practice.

Human beings always fall short of things because of life pressures. It could be stress pulling you down, it could be life provisions, it could be friends and families, and this means we do not need to be perfect every single time of our lives. When you fall today, this does not mean your end has come. You must strive to stand up again. You must find your way up again. These principles encourage you to gather your strength and stand up to your failures. It is a successful person falls so many time but makes sure he stands up to continue with the course. Only the quitters fall and never rise again, but the Reiki principles are giving you a chance to fall and rise to your feet again.

Just like when you wanted to know the multiplication table in the kindergarten, the teacher could make you sing it every day during the lesson so that it sinks in your mind and later you can interpret it yourself, this same process applies to the Reiki principles. If you want to know and understand the Reiki principles, you advised to say them out loud for at least two times.

To make it easier for you not to forget saying the Reiki principles, it is advisable that you print a big picture and place it where you can see it every day you go to the place the picture is hanged, or if you are a professional Reiki healer, you can hang the 5 principles of Reiki picture in your office or healing room so that each time you step in the principles are well displayed where you can see them and read them out.

All the Reiki principles are not the same. They are different from each other, and their perception can only be unlocked by a person using them. To be able to unlock the Reiki principle's perception, one has to meditate. Meditation gives the inner different view and understanding of what these Reiki principles mean. If you just read the Reiki principles out loudly every day two times, you might not be able to understand what they mean. They might become a song just like the kindergarten rhymes if one does not meditate to get the true reflection of the words in them. Your perception of Reiki might be very different from another person's perception, and this does not mean you are wrong, or he is wrong.

During your meditation time to gain your perception about the Reiki principles, you should close your eyes and repeat one principle for many times, making the principle your bottom line. In this time, allow your mind to move freely, let it float in every corner but make sure your consciousness is maintained. You should understand what is going on inside your body and your mind as you read the mantra, which is the principle. You will realize during the meditation time that different emotions will start flooding in; thoughts that you have never thought of will come knocking too. Some people decide to meditate in groups during this realization of Reiki principles. When you decide to do a group meditation, it is good to share each other's views and feelings after the exercise.

Below are the Reiki principles and how they work;

Just For Today, I Will Not Worry

When you are worried, a lot of stress comes in that brings a lot of imbalance in the body. The stress caused by your worrying cause s emotional imbalance that blocks the flow of energy in the body. When you want to handle a problem, you do not run away from the problem or let it pull you down. Worrying about a problem is not a solution; the solution is to embrace that problem. We should know that problems are there in life, and life does not have to be smooth always. There are ups and downs in life that we must face. We might not always be on the path we desire, but all these problems and setbacks should not weigh us down.

To overcome our worries will depend on how we react towards the worries because any responses directed to any worry decide on how we live our lives. Accepting that life is not smooth always and accepting the problems in life as opportunities, seeing the positivity of problems and utilizing this positivity will help us live a satisfying life. If we respond negatively to our worries, negative thoughts will come in, the body mind and soul balance will be distorted and stressing start haunting us which in the end will block the energy flow in the body and hinder any healing that is supposed to take place.

To reduce the worries in your life, allocate time to yourself. Find a time and do things that make you happy. You can go out to movies and laugh your heart out, you can invite friends to the house and watch a good movie and have fun talks that make you laugh, and you can read good funny magazines that will make you laugh. You can go swimming if it brings a lot of joy to you and makes the worries go away. It is said that laughter is the medicine of the heart, so when you laugh, you release the emotions from deep within that are worrying you and blocking your energy flow.

When this principle is unbalanced due to the worry affecting your life, you can be able to rebalance it by placing your hands on the root chakra and the heart chakra. Let your hands stay there as long as it is needed until you feel that they should be removed.

Just For Today, I Will Not Be Angry

Emotional effects on the body are not good because they cause the body to lose balance. Anger is an emotion that drains a lot of energy from the person it is directed to. Each time you get angry, all your control is lost. You cannot be able to think clearly, and your focus on important things becomes impaired. Your decision-making ability is reduced when you are angry, and you are bound to make so many mistakes that can be irreversible.

For us to get a remedy to anger, we first must know what brings it. What is that button that when it is pressed, gives all these emotional feelings? We should understand the trigger of anger before we can be able to manage it. In life generally, if you cannot understand the root cause of anything, you cannot be able to come up with solutions or preventive measure to the problem. This is not different here; understanding the trigger of anger will help you grasp a better solution or develop a preventive measure that will eliminate this anger or restrict it from affecting you or others.

When you are angry, you lose a lot of energy, and when others are angry, you drain them the energy. The other people or things that made you angry sucks the energy out of you, and you will not be able to control the energy flow at all. The balance in the body will be lost because energy drainage is high, and there is no good judgment and focus on its accumulation to perform the duties required.

When you understand how to manage your anger and control it, you can face any anger-driven issues that become your way. You will be able to understand every anger trigger and be able to remotely control them before they leave any effect to you or others. In any case, any person tries to press your anger trigger; you will simply look at it and smile because all the control is in your hands.

As much as anger is scaring when you do not know how to manage it, it is a choice. Everyone has a clear choice of whether to be angry or not to be angry. Restoration of balance to the body when it has failed due to anger, you must place your hand on the third eye chakra, and your other hand should be settled on the root chakra. This method will help you be able to get out all the emotions that are destroying the balance.

Just For Today, I Will Do My Work Honestly

When people hear about the word honest, everyone has his understanding. When you lie to get something from the office, and you think it did not matter, some will feel that it mattered a lot. For example, if you are a doctor working in the hospital and at the end of the day you decide to take some packs of painkillers from the office without permission to your house for your personal use, to you it may seem like nothing because you know the hospital has so many medicines. When another person looks at this scenario, he sees dishonesty in your work; there is theft in your work. You are stealing the medicines from your workplace, and it is not good.

You might have a talent that you need to use to benefit others, but if you do not use this talent and make sure it serves the right purpose, you will be dishonest in your work. You deny others the benefits they have to get from your talent, and you are also dishonest to yourself in that you deny yourself the chance to exercise this talent.

Honesty is inbuilt. It is a personality that someone has within his soul and mind, and it is not affected by whether people see it or not. Instead of wasting long hours in front of the television watching movies that will not help you, you should be using your time and talents honestly to help people that need them. Stop stealing the talent from you by denying it.

If the balance is lost due to being dishonest in your work, you can rebalance it by placing your hands on the third eye chakra and then on the solar plexus chakra and let the hands remain there until you feel that they no longer need to be there.

Just For Today, I Will Give Thanks To My Many Blessings

Sometimes life makes us feel that it is not fair, but we have to understand that life does not always give us what we want. Life only gives us what we need to survive. Our wants may be so many that if life decided to give everyone what they wanted, the balance in life would be completely lost. If you ever sang a song from the hymnbook that tells count your blessings name them one by one and you will be surprised what the Lord has done. This song is in the Christians hymn book; then you will understand that in life when you count all the blessings you have received, you will be surprised that there are so many. It is good to be grateful for what you have rather than complaining about what you have not achieved. A person who has legs without shoes should be grateful that at least they have legs unlike those who do not have legs they can put shoes on. Learn to look at the positive side of life and not dwelling on the negative only.

When you learn that you have to be grateful because of the good things in your life and decide to let go of all the negativity that materialistic things bring, you will be able to live a life of peace and joy.

Just For Today, I Will Be King to My Neighbor and Every Living Thing

Kindness is like computer data. There is terminology in the computer called garbage in garbage out. What you feed in is what you get. Kindness when you give it out, you will receive it. If you give out negativity, negativity will come right back to you. If the balance of this principle is disrupted, you can place your one hand on the third eye chakra then the other to the root chakra. Slowly move the hand from the third eye chakra to the throat chakra and the other hand from the root chakra to the heart chakra to restore the balance.

Chapter 12: Heal Your Emotional And Mental Health

Mindfulness

Historically in the reiki tradition, the use of mindfulness is absolutely necessary even beginning in the first degree of training, but it is emphasized even more so in the second degree, due to the intense nature of training in the advanced level. So what exactly is mindfulness? It is being conscious and aware during the present moment. That moment may last as long as a single breath, it may last for a full hour of meditation, or it may be something you strive for in every waking moment of your life. Because our lives are only made up of a collection of individual breaths, there is no better way to celebrate and appreciate your life more fully than by being conscious of each one of those. What has already happened is no longer your life. It is gone. I hope you appreciated it. What will happen is not your life. It is a creation of your imagination. Don't you want a life even better than you can possibly imagine? Then do not waste your time imagining so small. Exist in the here and now and you will experience it when it comes.

It is important to note that mindfulness is not an end goal to arrive at, but instead it a practice that leads you on a journey for however long you want to be on it. There is no failing at mindfulness; it is more about the effort to try. A crucial part of the practice is to come back to mindfulness after falling off track. Whether that means breathing mindfully, getting lost in thought, and then coming back to the breath, or if that means stopping yourself mid-word when you realize you are about to say something negative or that you might regret. These are all ways that you practice coming back to mindfulness, and in fact, is not a failure of mindfulness, but rather a part of its success.

Just like so many things we are discussing in this book, it is a skill that you must practice in order to improve upon. And just like reiki, it is something that all of us already have and possess. There is only teaching about it in order to channel it. It is something that absolutely everyone can--and should!--do. It is accessible to everyone, and the benefits are enormous. Because it is a natural and instantly gratifying act, it takes little to no extra knowledge or effort to apply it. And because you are simply applying it to the life you already live, it does not necessarily take any time out of your schedule, planning, or special accommodations to include it. Nor does mindfulness require that you commit to some huge life change or acceptance that something in your life is wrong. Quite the contrary, in fact. A key tenet of mindfulness is that you accept and come to terms with exactly the truth of the moment, without any type of judgement at all. There are no comparisons as to what is right or wrong, good or bad, or choosing what needs improvements. There is simply the deeply contentedness of acceptance.

Because the act of being present in the moment is a difficult challenge, especially at first, it will take some practice before you are able to be mindful for more than a fleeting moment at a time. That is quite all right. But you will notice, the more you practice, the easier it becomes and the longer those moments will last.

As a reiki practitioner, mindfulness should become a way of life for you. Again, it is not necessary that you are perfect at it and never fall off track. In fact, if you were able to be totally mindful at all times, you may just be considered to be the second coming of Buddha. Short of that, that makes you a mere mortal like the rest of us, and perfection is not necessary. According to some, the simple act of being mindful, present, and aware of each moment is considered the absolute meaning of life. This means that each thought you have, each movement you make, each intention you set is done so with a consciousness and determination that imparts an almost spiritual-level of support behind it. It means that in every moment you are accepting of what is. You are not ruminating in the past. You are not worrying about the future. You are not wishing that things were different. You are not upset by things that you cannot change. You are not reactionary to outside stimuli. You are not swept away by your emotions.

All of that being said, you might have noticed that mindfulness sounds a lot like the amount of attention it takes to practice reiki. That is exactly correct! Mindfulness and reiki go hand-in-hand; not because they are the same thing, but because they utilize the same kind of "muscles." While it is amazingly beneficial, it is not necessary that you sit in meditation in order to perform reiki. In fact, reiki is a type of mindfulness, because you are focusing on the life source coursing through the Earth and your body. Applying the conscious thought is absolutely crucial to the art of healing by laying hands because while you are doing so, you cannot be focused on the results of your healing, how great you will feel after, or what you expect to happen as a result of it. These are all manifestations of your ego and are future focused. That will distract from the mindfulness and make your reiki less effective. There is no predicted outcome of any session, and to attempt to imagine the outcome is a form of pride in the face of the power of the unimaginable Universe's power.

Instead, when performing reiki, either on yourself or another, it is of the utmost importance that you filter out all nonessential thoughts and expectations of what you are doing and what it might bring. The placing of your hands should happen with a clear mind, and that will assist in the blissful feeling of being one with the Universe. Allowing yourself to give over fully to the power of the original life source is the ultimate moment of mindfulness. It is the moment you will be most effective in channeling the Earth's energy, because you have fully removed yourself from the process. You are completely one with and in service to the life source.

Mental and Emotional Healing

One of the many benefits of using reiki is to heal our mental health. This level of healing, however, requires being a second-degree student of the art. This area of healing is where we focus and are able to work with the conscious level of our thought process. Through this level we can recognize, alter, and improve upon our judgements, patterns, habits, and behaviors.

Because, as was discussed with performing reiki on others, reiki only applies as much healing as is necessary and the person is ready and willing to accept, this means that you cannot heal your mental health any more than you are ready to. So although it seems nice, you will not be able to become a second-degree reiki student and instantly become enlightened. It will still be a gradual process that occurs with each new step of growth along the way.

There should be no concern over the efficacy or security of healing your own or anyone else's mental health, because as has been discussed in previous chapters, it cannot be manipulated for negative purposes. It does not resemble or act like any type of dark manipulation like hypnosis or spells. Again, it is merely the life source of the Universe correcting an imbalance, even in a mental capacity.

If you are interested in working with your mental wellbeing in general, you can do so by simply focusing your energy on a mental level. No need to have a specific goal in mind or challenge to overcome, but the mere act of channeling the life energy to improving your mental health will accomplish this. Through reiki you are activating the efforts and "muscles" of self-improvement, introspection, mindfulness, and self-care to encourage energy flow through these areas of your life. Much like physical exercise, creating a routine is crucial in building up your effectiveness and outcomes, even in reiki. Through repeated mental focus of energy you will be more able to recognize patterns that you have, conscious or unconscious, reflect upon how those patterns are serving you, decide if that is something you want to change, and then brainstorm how and why you would change that.

You can also focus on specific problems in your mental capacity. This will require a clear understanding of exactly what you are trying to work through in order to best focus your energy there. The amazing thing about reiki is, although you may notice an area you want to change, you do not have to know exactly how to change it or what the solution is. Because reiki provides exactly what is needed in exactly the way it can be best accepted at that time, the Universe's knowledge will be all that you need. You can help channel more energy by using tools like the symbols mentioned in chapter one; you will need to become a second-degree reiki practitioner to learn how to best activate these triggers. You can also combine these tools with the use of chanting, affirmations, or mantras. All of these can be done either silently inside your mind, or you can say them aloud. Either will work, but studies show that there is an extra element of healing vibrations that occur within yourself when you speak or chant aloud.

To become advanced in your reiki practice, it actually requires a certain level of mental healing in this way. Because the channeling and focusing of the Universe's energy requires a certain level of enlightenment and connection with the Universe, this cannot be done with a closed mind. You must begin any reiki practice with a certain level of self-awareness in order to harness the life force. One cannot possibly humble themselves enough to attempt to sue the original source energy of the world without this base level of mental aptitude and introspection necessary to heal one's own mind. The focus of our energy is reflected and manifested in our thoughts. Therefore, the more in control and focused your mind is, the more in control and focused your energy practice will be.

The Rules of Reiki

There are generally five accepted rules to follow in order to get your mind the proper place for reiki. These are general tenets that, much like mindfulness, are more about the journey of attempting them, rather than subscribing successfully to them at all times.

Today only, I will...

Not be moved to anger.

Not worry.

Humble myself.

Work honestly.

Use compassion in all that I do.

Today only, I will...

To begin with, all of the guidelines begin with the phrase, "Today only, I will..." in order to serve as a reminder of our mindfulness practice. The only time to focus on is the moment happening right now, and therefore, when it comes to our guiding principles, it only makes sense to focus on what is in our control, which is today only. To set a goal that is too grand or too large to accomplish will only serve to discourage you from attempting it. If a task seems too insurmountable to be completed, at the first sign of difficulty, you will have no reason to pick yourself, dust yourself off, and give it another try. Rather, these guidelines are built to do the opposite; they give you the very small, very manageable goal of not worrying about any other day. Not worrying about any streak of days going unbroken. Not worrying about cheat days or weekends. No, with these guidelines, you only have to focus on following them today. Yesterday is gone and tomorrow you can do whatever you want. Just worry about trying these things today.

Not be moved to anger.

Anger is a reactionary emotion. Anger is not something one comes to after a lot of thought. It bubbles up inside of you uncontrollably, trying to take over our nervous system, our energy, our thoughts, and our reasoning. That is why the first tenant is to do our best to overcome this. We cannot experience life at our highest energy vibration if we are stuck in anger. This emotion usually arises from a disconnect between what you want to be happening and what is actually happening. Fortunately for all of us, we cannot control everything--or much of anything--so this is a responsibility we should take off our own plate. Think about it like this: to be angry about something that you cannot control is the ultimate example of fruitlessness. That is a lot of energy spent on nothing.

2. Not worry.

Worry is an emotion based in another time. Either you are worried about something in the past that has already happened that you cannot change, or you are worried about something in the future that has not happened and that you cannot change. Both of these instances mean you are not living in the present moment, which is the only time that matters, and is the only time that is applicable to reiki healing.

3. Humble myself.

To be grateful is to be humble. You cannot fully appreciate the gifts that are given to you if you fancy yourself so important that occurrences are rendered a nuisance. For that reason, you should try to humble yourself in order to utilize the massive force that is reiki and be grateful for the energy flowing through you.

4. Work honestly.

Integrity means doing the right thing all the time, even when you will not get noticed or recognition for doing so. It is that little voice inside of you telling you when you are veering off course, and it will not let you settle until you get right with it. To work honestly means that your integrity is in line with your conscious, telling you that you can sleep easy knowing you did your best. Truly, the only way to learn and become better is to be honest about where you are, where you want to go, and how you are progressing.

The Universe does not have time for your ego-stroking illusions. It only knows and cares about the truth, so you should meet it on its level.

5. Use compassion in all that I do.

The ultimate requirement in reiki is to have compassion. The life force energy that we are attempting to manipulate unites us with every other thing in the Universe. That means we truly are all one. The only way to use reiki is positively, and the easiest way to feel the love and understanding you share with others is by showing them compassion. To honor and respect every other being's journey, struggles, triumphs, and energy is the most holy thing a human can do, and that is what reiki asks of all of us.

Chapter 13: Imagination Playtime (It's Not Just For Kids)

Learning to use your imagination to help you focus your concentration is the next step toward learning Reiki. Yes, it's time to play with your imagination!

Interestingly enough, you actually use your imagination more often than you probably think. You know all those nagging little doubts you have about yourself, others or things you hear about? Even that skepticism you felt when you first started reading this book about Reiki? That's your imagination thinking up all the possible outcomes of a single, simple thought.

You probably know how to use your imagination, but allow me to walk you through the steps I think will make it easier for you to focus.

Find a place that is quiet and free of distractions and sit or lay down so that you are comfortable, but not likely to fall asleep. Now close your eyes and clear your mind as much as you can from outside distractions and thoughts for what you need to do later on in your day.

Concentrate and remember what a pot of boiling water looks like. You don't have to think about the stove it is on, just the pot and the water boiling inside. It's okay if you can't see the image clearly in your mind but the more clearly you can reconstruct the image, the more defined your focus will be.

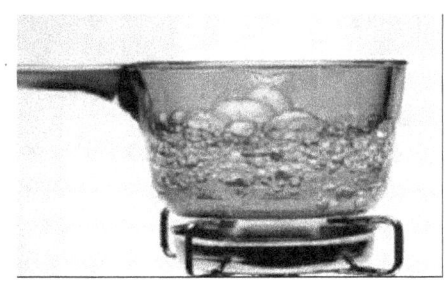

Do you see something in your mind? It may be flat or fuzzy, maybe a bit wobbly around the edges but that is perfectly fine. As long as you see something, you're doing great!

Once you have that image in your mind, the next step is to make it better, firm up the outline and bring it into better focus. You can do this by really thinking about it and bring the details back to your memory.

What is the color of the part that holds the water?

Make the pot in your mind the color you remember.

Is the pot glass or metal?

Does it have a texture on the outside surface of the pot? Are there any grooves, decorative enameling or is it completely smooth? Is it dull, shiny or something in between?

What about the handle or handles of the pot. Does it have a single handle? Is it plastic, glass, metal or silicone?

What shape is the handle? How thick is it? Are there any grooves in the handle to make it easy to hold? Is it riveted, welded or molded to the bowl of the pot?

Once you feel like you have remembered everything you can about that pot of water, open your eyes and look at the world around you. Just let your mind wander for a few minutes and let those synapses relax a little.

Let's expand on this exercise. Close your eyes. Bring everything you remember about your pot back to mind and sharpen that image in your memory. Can you see it? Does it look like you could reach out and touch it? You're doing very well! Now imagine more details to the picture in your mind.

How much water is in the pot? Is it halfway up the side or just an inch below the rim?

Is it boiling fast or slow?

Can you imagine the sound of the water boiling?

What does the boiling water smell like?

Can you feel the heat radiating off the pot?

This is the step that will probably take you the longest in which to become proficient. Once you have that pot of boiling water pictured in your mind, you need to fix it in your mind so that you can call it up whenever you want. You can do that by describing it in vivid detail to someone else, recording it with a tape recorder, typing it out in a word-processing document or writing it down in a journal.

Most people can commit things to memory when they do three things with the information: see or read it, write it down, and hear it. This is why teachers will have power points up on a screen while they are giving a lecture and the student is taking notes. The student sees the words or pictures on the power point, they hear the instructor's words and they write those words down, allowing them to commit the lesson to memory. When you can listen to or read your description and picture it in your mind with no trouble, then you know the description is good.

Now that your description is vivid, you can go on to the next step of focusing. Bring your image to mind. You should be able to hear the water gurgling in the pot, the sound of the pot contracting or expanding as temperature changes occur and any sounds the heat source makes like the soft hiss of the gas flowing to fuel the flames on a gas stove or a slight ticking as electricity heats an element on an electric stove.

Imagine yourself leaning over the pot. You should be able to look into the pot and see the water boiling and the steam rising from the roiling surface. Breathe the steam in.

How does it smell?

Can you taste the metallic flavor of the chemical treatment of the water being released?

You should be able to feel the difference in temperature as the steam rises to touch your face.

Feel the gentle pressure of the steam as it causes your skin to react to its presence.

Feel the moisture from the steam in your sinuses and maybe your lungs.

Excellent! It isn't completely necessary to imagine the pot of boiling water in this detail but the better you can see it, the easier it will be for you to use and utilize Reiki. This exercise will really help you to visualize the streams of energy flowing into and through your body.

You may still be skeptical about actually being able to see or feel this energy since most people consider energy as being without substance. Substance, as in something that can be felt and seen like the steam rising from your pot of boiling water, is energy that can be seen and felt.

What does this energy look like? It is different for each person who practices Reiki. There are many ways that the energy can look to you. You may see it as a distortion of color like oil on wet pavement, or a cloud of color like seeing something bright through a sheet of water. It might just be a spot of color brighter than anything around it.

What does this energy feel like? Again, there are so many ways that the body can interpret the sensations given off by this energy that it is nearly impossible to tell you how you will feel it. It may be a simple change in temperature, usually warmer but sometimes cooler. You might feel a change in pressure against your skin. It might tingle, though not painfully as when your foot or hand falls asleep. You might experience it as a vibration or even a sound. It might be a simple tone or a low or high harmonic tone. It may sound like a chant or song with both melody and harmony making it a collection of sounds. However you experience this energy, believe that you really did see, feel or hear what you saw, felt or heard.

Expanding your senses

Now that you've experienced this energy, let's go back to your pot of boiling water. Once you have that image in your mind, add some rice to the boiling water. Let it cook! See the rice grains moving in the water as they start to absorb the water. You can almost see how the bubbles form and roll to the surface to break and release a puff of steam. Lean in and smell the steam now. Do you remember how wonderful cooking rice smells?

Take a clean, clear glass and hold it in the steam. Watch as the steam condenses on the glass and makes it cloudy. Take the glass away and let the steam evaporate. The glass isn't clean anymore, is it? There is a film that dulls the clear glass. This is because some of the rice actually gets carried away with the steam and gives it that lovely smell. Rice is food or nutrition for your body. If you don't get enough nourishment, you will find it difficult to function properly and can become malnourished. Becoming malnourished can lead to illness that causes your body to malfunction and can even lead to death if it continues for too long. Getting the proper nutrition allows your body to function properly and makes it possible for you to live.

Consider that metaphor. Don't think about it, experience it. Let it fill your mind as you concentrate on every aspect of it: see it, smell it, hear it and feel it. Make it so real in your mind that you can reach out and touch it. Then learn from what you see.

This game of imagination will help you to focus your concentration just as feeling your breathing helped you center yourself. These are the beginning steps of learning to use Reiki and are a form of meditation in and of themselves. They will be used to allow you to enter into a relaxed state that encourages the flow of the life force energy through your body and takes care of those ripples and knots from the lines of energy that run throughout your body or someone else.

The next step to learning how to use Reiki and that life force energy is pretty fun and relaxing. Take a look and enjoy!

Chapter 14: Reiki And Also The Mood

We could see in Quantum physics defines deep space as power with power as well as concern being compatible. In Psychology, Eastern Philosophies, Holistic medicine as well as Faith of Numerous typical cultures, they all have terms for the word "life" indicating power.

The mood is a power area bordering the physical body. In ordinary terms, the mood is a power area that borders the physical body yet the majority of individuals do not see it unless they have a present to do so with the nude eye. In importance the mood is an electro-magnetic area that borders the human physical body or HEF (human power area) as well as every microorganism and also item in the universe.

The Psychological or Important auric physical body- The psychological physical body is egg designed and also consists of the various other 2. The psychological physical body is likewise linked to our previously, which could trigger troubles. It is crucial to discover just how to manage various feelings throughout a day, the threat is or else that they come to be subdued as well as saved in the psychological physical body and also could later on be the reason of clogs as well as disruptions leading to clinical issues.

Psychological Physical body or Celestial Psychological Physical body- This auric physical body offers to instruct us self-knowledge. The psychological physical body as its name indicates mirrors the mindful mind, reasoning, intelligence as well as energetic reasoning. It is this auric degree that allows us to have caring partnerships with household and also buddies.

The Etheric Theme Physical body (Divine Will)/ Reduced psychological auric physical body- This houses the divine will certainly we all bring within us. The Etheric Design template likewise saves the existing and also all the feasible futures. It is attached to the Throat chakra.

The Holy or Greater Psychological Auric Physical body- This auric degree mirrors the subconscious mind that is a component of the non-active component of our human brain. This physical body is connected with Magnificent love, as well as spiritual euphoria. It is linked to the Third eye chakra.

The Causal physical body (Ketheric Theme) or the Spiritual Instinctive Physical body- The powers in this physical body rotates with a quite high regularity. This is where the spirit connects with the aware mind using the subconscious mind in the psychological physical body. It is this auric physical body that attaches to divine mind and also to comprehend the higher global pattern.

Offer on your own Reiki for an only a few mins. You could call them after that to see just what they experienced and also discuss just what you noticed.

Finish with thankfulness for the present of Reiki.

A number of our desires could be discovered in the etheric physical body. With the help of rules, signs, importance and so on one could impact the feature of this component of the mood. Linked to the Origin chakra.

Each Chakra as well as Auric Physical body has a Shade that Represents it as it sends out light.

RED MOOD SHADE: Connects to the physique, heart or flow. The densest shade, it produces one of the most rubbing. Rubbing brings in or wards off; cash fears or fascinations; rage or ruthless; anxiousness or anxiety

Crimson: Grounded, sensible, energetic, solid will-power, survival-oriented.

Muddied red: Temper (driving away).

Clear red: Powerful, energetic, affordable, sex-related, enthusiastic.

Pink-bright as well as light: Caring, tender, delicate, sensuous, imaginative, love, pureness, empathy; brand-new or revitalized enchanting partnership. Could suggest clairaudience.

Dark as well as dirty pink: Immature and/or unethical nature.

Orange Red: Self-confidence, innovative power.

In an excellent, brilliant and also pure state, red power could act as a healthy and balanced ego.

ORANGE MOOD SHADE: Connects to reproductive body organs and also feelings. The shade of vigor, vitality, healthiness as well as exhilaration. Great deals of power as well as endurance, imaginative, efficient, bold, brave, outbound social nature; presently experiencing anxiety pertaining to hungers and also dependencies;.

Orange-Yellow: Creative, smart, information oriented, nit-picker, clinical.

Chapter 15: What Is Energy Healing?

What is energy? What is energy healing? Can everyone benefit from energy healing? These are some of the questions I will answer as you follow along. It has become more prevalent in recent years with the rise of alternative remedies due to the ever-growing frustration with traditional medicine.

Energy healing is a natural form of alternative medicine that has its roots in ancient Eastern and Western cultures. It's prevalent in the Americas, Asia, India, and Egypt. Energy healing is a method of healing that manipulates the subtle energies of the body to heal the mind, body, and spirit. Practitioners believe that when the energy is out of alignment in the body, we may become ill due to obstructions in the flow of energy.

Asian countries, such as China and Japan, have created a medical system based on energy levels in the body. In Traditional Chinese Medicine (TCM), this energy that is within us all is known as CHI. This energy, or chi, in our bodies has a holistic or whole-body impact, meaning it affects our physical, emotional, and spiritual health. Energy healing seeks to remove obstructions in the body to allow energy to flow freely, thus ensuring good health.

Roots of Reiki

Reiki is a spiritual energy healing art form created in Japan thousands of years ago, but it didn't emerge in popularity until the late 1800s. The modern form of Reiki was developed in 1922 by a Japanese Buddhist named Mikao Osui, teaching over 2000 students in his lifetime. The practice then spread to America via Hawaii in the 1940s, then to Europe in the 1980s. Reiki comes from the Japanese words REI, meaning "universal life" or "higher power", and KI, meaning "energy" or "life force." This practice of healing energy involves the transfer of universal energy through the palms of the practitioner to the patient. Sometimes it is referred to as palm healing or hands-on healing. There is some controversy around Reiki (and most alternative treatments) because they have not been studied and backed by scientific data. However, a 2007 study shows that around 1.2 million people in America have tried Reiki or similar healing energy therapies in the previous year, proving its immense popularity. Numerous hospitals across the U.S. and Europe, meanwhile, are offering Reiki and healing energy alternative therapies to their patients.

While Reiki is a spiritual practice, it does not have its roots in any one religion, and it has no dogma or special set of beliefs. Because Reiki comes from God, or the divine creator, Reiki can help people get more in touch with their religion, but Reiki in and of itself is not a religious belief. However, Reiki masters do promote a life of harmony with others to promote peace within one's own life, which is the basis for most religions. Reiki is the life force that flows through all living things. Your energy, chi, or ki, should be free-flowing and strong, which in turn promotes good health. Osui is credited for rediscovering the root system that is now called Reiki, and his methods and traditions have been passed down through grandmasters over the years. Osui also created a model for Reiki called the Reiki Ideals, who based them on the five principles of the Meiji emperor whom Osui admired. The ideals in English are translated thusly:

The secret art of inviting happiness.

The miraculous medicine of all diseases.

Just for today, do not anger.

Do not worry and be filled with gratitude.

Devote yourself to your work.

Be kind to people.

Every morning and evening, join your hands in prayer.

Pray these words to your heart

and chant these words with your mouth.

Osui designed the Ideals to create a spiritual balance within Reiki. Their purpose is to help people realize that healing the spirit by consciously resolving to improve upon ourselves is a necessary part of Reiki healing. In order for Reiki healing to have lasting results, we must accept responsibility for our healing, and take a proactive part in it.

Today, the Usui System of Natural Healing is the most widely used form of Reiki. Practitioners and teachers are trained through an initiation process where the knowledge of Reiki is passed down through Reiki masters. Anyone can learn Reiki, as it is not dependent upon one's intelligence or level of spirituality. It is not taught in the traditional sense, as the knowledge of Reiki is "transferred" to the student during a Reiki class. These abilities are passed on from master to student through an "attunement" which is the process of becoming attuned, or aware, of the energy inside of us. The student is able to tap into a never-ending supply of life force energy to improve health and well-being, which can then be shared with others.

Reiki is a healing technique that takes away our stress and illnesses through the "laying on" of hands. Reiki is a simple, safe, and natural process that can help almost every known physical, mental, or spiritual malady. A treatment feels like a warm light flowing through your body that promotes feelings of peace, tranquility, security, and well-being. It also works with traditional medicine to relieve side effects and promote quicker recovery.

Chapter 16: How Is Healing Expected To Be Obtained From Using This Medication Techniques?

Rebalances Chakras

The capacity of Reiki to rebalance the chakras gives creative advantages to another slate. While promoting the self-confidence needed for unbridled speech, chakras that are balanced and spinning merrily improve the link to creative energies. By invigorating and unifying the body, mind, and spirit, all types of creativity can blossom fully. Dancers are able to dance more freely, painters are able to paint more deeply, and authors can write more deeply.

Quiets the Monkey Mind

In the creative process or any process for that matter, the restless, relentless chatter of the mind can bring a large dent. Reiki can take care of it, calming the constant stream of fear, self-doubt, and other intrusive thoughts of the mind. Once the mind is quiet, from a powerful and grounded base, you can explore the universe much easier.

Reiki Sensations

As Reiki energies flow throughout the Reiki session between the physician and the recipient, the two bodies may respond or react with specific sensations. These feelings are almost always enjoyable. You may feel heat, warmth, cold, subtlety, stamina, or strength. The fact that you can feel that Reiki flows, whether you give it or receive it, is to verify that the energy is being welcomed.

What Reiki Feels Like

Reiki experience is as distinctive as everyone who receives Reiki. People have recorded common sensations such as feeling heat or coolness, tingling, vibration or noise, itchiness and/or somnolence. During the meeting, some individuals reported "feeling" nothing physical but after the session was over, they noticed beneficial modifications.

Reiki operates like a body regulating the thermostat. Like a furnace that switches on and off automatically to control the temperature, Reiki flows slowly or quickly, as needed, to dispense balancing energies. Reiki sometimes moves erratically, sometimes smoothly, like a pendulum swinging back and forth.

Using Reiki to Help with a Career Change

Whether you're fed up, burned out, or just finally gathered the confidence to call it quits at your current job, your cards may have a career change. And if you use Reiki to assist you both target your dream job and set you up for achievement, you have a nice opportunity to play those cards right. While it can be an interesting prospect to change careers, it is also one that can take an avalanche of stress and fear just as rapidly. Leaving your ancient job behind and its safety can begin the engine of stress and fear, which turns into complete gear when you start bombarding your mind with a host of issues:

Should I go for something that I enjoy or make me wealthy? What if this fresh career bored me?

Does anybody even hire?

What kind of training, training, and abilities do I need? Will I create sufficient cash to survive?

What if I completely mess it up and end up breaking up, living alone and somewhere on the side of a highway?

Improve This with Letting Go and Letting Higher Energy Flow

For performers, additional blocks may include fear of making a mistake, perfectionism, or otherwise becoming so strongly invested in a project's outcome that they are too paralyzed to even make the first step. Reiki can increase creativity by promoting relaxation by assisting you to let go of the result, the need to perfect, the paralyzing fear, and other barriers that may hinder the creative process. You are more easily able to link with your intuition when your resistance to letting go and being your true self is relinquished. You can also let something greater shine through than yourself. You can be open to the beautiful instead of attempting to manage your creative output.

Letting Go of the "I"

Reiki's entire scheme is about letting go of the "I".

This was noted out very obviously by Mikao Usui within the precepts:

- Don't be upset.
- Don't be afraid.
- Be thankful.
- Do this conscientiously.

- Show yourself and others kindness.

If we only look at the precepts at a superficial level, we won't see that they're about letting go of the "I," but if we look more deeply into them, we can see that clearly. Let's ask some questions for ourselves and see what the responses are.

Who gets worried? I get worried. Who's getting upset? I'm getting upset.

Who wouldn't be thankful? I'm not thankful.

Who's sympathetic in the manner? I'm sympathetic in my manner.

Who is not diligently practicing? I'm not in the manner of diligent practice.

Reiki Precepts – A Deeper Perspective

Looking deeper into it, we can slowly start to see that this is why the precepts are about letting go of the "I." If we let go of the "I," then there is no "I" that gets angry or worried. In the way of being grateful, not living diligently, or being compassionate, there is no "I."

It seems, however, that we often try to strengthen the grip on the "I" in many Reiki system doctrines, rather than gradually (and maybe one day completely) letting go of the "I." Looking at an example of other hands-on healing.

When we feel something while doing practical healing on others, we often begin labeling what we feel; for instance, we may feel something and label it heat. We could say to ourselves as quickly as we label it heat; "because I feel the heat, I need to use this symbol now." Or we could say: "because I feel the heat this means my client has a severe problem."

Labeling, distinguishing, and judging all come from the "I"

Labeling, distinguishing and judging all come from the "I" –I feel this and so I'm going to do it to my customer. Apart from being "doing" rather than "being," we tighten our grip on the "I" by labeling, distinguishing and judging. So we can also ask some easy questions for ourselves: Who is labeling? Who distinguishes? Who is it that judges? The response to all these questions is "I am."

Been Mindful

In his teaching, Mikao Usui also added methods of mindfulness, such as Joshin Kokyu Ho, or focused on a mantra or symbol. "Awareness needs observation, but it must be free from interpretation and judgment." -Tarthang Tulku These methods of awareness are also there to assist us to let go of the "I" so that we can achieve the ultimate teachings within the Reiki scheme: Just be.

Simply be.

When we're just simply being with our client, we begin to enter a state of unity that can't occur when the "I" is engaged. Because once there's an "I," there's an "I" and "you" and suddenly we're distinct.

Being Reiki is the essence of the teachings of Mikao Usui, but to be alone we must let go of the "I." QUESTION: Does letting go of the "I" mean we're losing our distinctive humanity

— say, our beliefs, our lovely singing voice, our chocolate ice cream love? And when we go through our lives, become a bland, nameless, faceless individual with no views?

No; it just implies that we're letting go of attachments to ideas like, "I'm more aged and experienced than you because I've been practicing for 5 years and you've just begun," "My voice is more enjoyable to listen to than yours because I've got an ideal pitch," or "I have a more advanced palate than you because I like chocolate and you like vanilla." While each of these–compare, label, distinguish, judge–may be true to our human minds, they all believe.

Separateness is a cloud.

And secretly holding on to "I" and "you" — is like attempting to hold on to a cloud, something that is going to come and go temporarily. If instead we practice "free of interpretation and passing judgment" consciousness, if we practice Reiki's system in this way, we can begin to loosen our grip on the "I" and hold on to something that has always been and is with us, our True Self. We can just Be.

Chapter 17: Learning To Practice Reiki

Reiki (affirmed 'beam keep') is normally seen to be (just) a type of spiritual healing. However Reiki is more than this: Reiki is presently also increasingly viewed as a confidence and conduct approach towards individual satisfaction, whose principles and rationality can explain and accomplish better life-adjust and well-being; empower the furthering of self-improvement and discovery, and in addition being an exceptional healing and recovery treatment. Taking into account extremely ancient Eastern teachings, Reiki methodology and history has offered rise to perplexity, hypothesis and secret, in spite of the fact that lately, joyfully, the consistency and subtle element of information about Reiki has logically enhanced, to the point today where Reiki is an acknowledged type of 'option therapy', accessible and rehearsed generally, including its proposal and provision by numerous "mainstream" hospitals and clinics over the western world.

Reiki information and principles are especially deserving of inclusion in this online asset on account of their pertinence to self-improvement, well-being, to our understanding of mind and body, and how our minds are associated with the universe around us. The Reiki idea and its underpinning theory therefore give a superb point of view to improving energy about the mind-body link, and the principles of life-adjust and well-being. The majority of the substance of this article, and the brief for me to concentrate on this fascinating subject, has been given by Reiki Master and writer, Katharina Van Gent, which is appreciatively recognized.

Other regular wonders we have come to make them understand of include: gravity, magnetism, plate tectonics and quantum material science, also enormous advances in physical brain capacity and brain research.

In this way, to come back to our "inadequate" faculties: despite the fact that our reality gives off an impression of being still and strong, we now understand that truth be told everything is moving, and at a sub-nuclear level, everything is a long way from strong. Actually everything has extraordinary holes in the middle of the particles. The core of a particle is the main really thick piece of it - incredibly the extent of the core in connection to the measure of the molecule is similar to a pea in a show corridor. Electrical charge is really in charge of solidity, not density or solidity of molecules, which are for the most part purge space.

And everything vibrates at its own recurrence. Through the devoted work of scientists in numerous disciplines we have gone to a scientific affirmation of what psychically sensitive people have long-term held: There is more going on in the universe than our limited faculties can see, albeit a few people appear pre-disposed to tune into and somehow, understand this vitality. Maybe it is because of this scientific meticulousness that integral types of healing and option methods for understanding our reality, are increasingly being given recognition as being deserving of genuine consideration.

Reiki is presently part of an overall development of people who are legitimately worried about their welfare and their friends and family - and indeed the planet. People are seeking to assume liability for their own particular health, working with routine medicine yet extending those limits. Admitting that people are simply part of a nature structure may appear to be diminishing at in the first place, however truth be told it is empowering on the grounds that understanding the standards of the amusement (how the structure works) empowers one to utilize it to individual favorable position and to help other people. It becomes us to teach ourselves; challenge the 'got wisdom' (with generosity of spirit); investigate new thoughts; allow the outcomes of our enterprises; and regard every experience as possibly something from which we can develop.

Identified with this it is useful to consider a Japanese idea known as "tastemaker" which (despite the fact that on a literal level is a service for putting the structure in a Japanese house) also, and all the more pertinently, speaks to the maintenance of an agreeably adjusted society. This reasoning of 'promoting useful for all' is found in other societies and convictions too, and as a positive, giving, widely inclusive methodology serves both as a critical driver, and connection, for Reiki's qualities and points.

The mind-body association

The thought that all life is somehow basically different manifestations of an incredible life power can be found in religious and philosophical writings from all ages and societies. Psychologist Sigmund Freud's protégé, Carl Yung composed of an 'aggregate oblivious' as did Boris Pasternak (acclaimed Russian creator of Dr. Chicago), and this tract from Buddhist content is another case:

Feathered winged creatures and fishes finned

And mists and rain and quiet and wind

And sun and moon and stars say

All life is one life everywhere.

It is no more controversial when scientists from different disciplines guarantee that everything vibrates and despite appearances in actuality, is interconnected by some so far incomprehensible power and thus, to some degree, everything affects everything else.

Since this 'everything' must include contemplations, and musings are an emerging quality of the brain, and the brain is a piece of the body/individual - (would you be able to see where this is leading) - it stands to reason that present day medicine too, is looking again at integral therapies and spiritual/common healing to perceive how it accommodates with this new understanding.

That 'the mind influences the body and the body influences the mind' has for some time been acknowledged in the realm of option/integral therapy. It appears that this ancient idea is being affirmed by today's science.

And this is where Reiki comes in. Reiki just takes advantage of this infinite vitality for the mental and physical well-being of both the practitioner and beneficiary. The Reiki practitioner is only a conduit through whom the vitality streams into the beneficiary, and the practitioner has the glad point of interest of benefiting from the session too...

Conclusion

The Reiki treatment is both beneficial and rewarding to practitioner and a recipient's. It is always unique and no explanation can really explain the amazement that the experience can inspire. It is a pleasure to both treat and receive Reiki. The deeper you work with Reiki and the more it flows.

www.ingramcontent.com/pod-product-compliance
Lightning Source LLC
Chambersburg PA
CBHW072014070526
44583CB00015B/1476